The funky fresh juice book

Jason Vale
Juice Master

V2

For all your juicy needs simply go to...

www.juicemaster.com

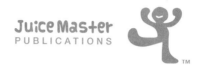

First published in 2011 by Juice Master Publications.

Updates and Reprinted 2013 by Juice Master Publications.

Copyright © Jason Vale & Juice Master Publications 2013.

ISBN 978-0-9547664-1-2

Written by Jason Vale with acknowledged contributions.

Photography by Kris Talikowski, Jason Vale, Kate Beswick, Ordinary Toucan LLP, Gareth Cattermole/Getty Images Entertainment (page 161), Ryan Pierse/Getty Images Sport (page 163).

Design & layout by Ordinary Toucan LLP

Printed and bound by Butler Tanner and Dennis Limited.

Printed on FSC certified paper.

While the author of this book has made every effort to ensure that the information contained in this book is as accurate and up-to-date as possible at the time of publication, medical and pharmaceutical knowledge is constantly changing and the application of it to particular circumstances depends on many factors. This book should not be used as an alternative to specialist medical advice and it is recommended that readers always consult a qualified medical profession for individual advice before following any new diet or health programme. The author and the publishers cannot be held responsible for any errors and omissions that can be found in the text, or any actions that may be taken by a reader, as a result of any reliance on the information contained in the text, which are taken entirely at the reader's own risk.

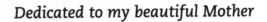

Dedicated to my beautiful Mother

I was the luckiest man alive
to have had you in my life.

You were my best-friend,
my teacher, my mentor, my world.

The world is a poorer place without
you in it but your legacy lives on.

I promised I would continue with the mission of
helping as many people as possible – and I will.

You always told me "Turn your lemons into lemonade,"
and I will continue to do that on every level.

I still cannot quite believe you will never read this...
I miss you every single day and I cannot thank you
enough for being my mother, I was blessed beyond
words... Rest in peace wherever you are.

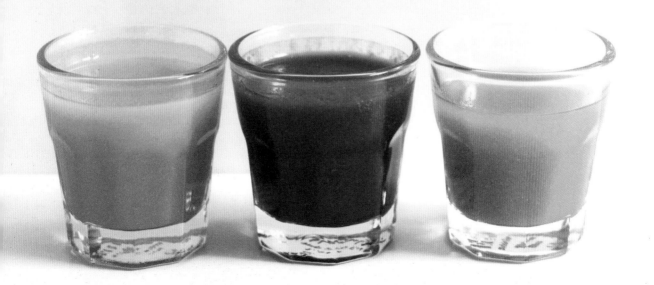

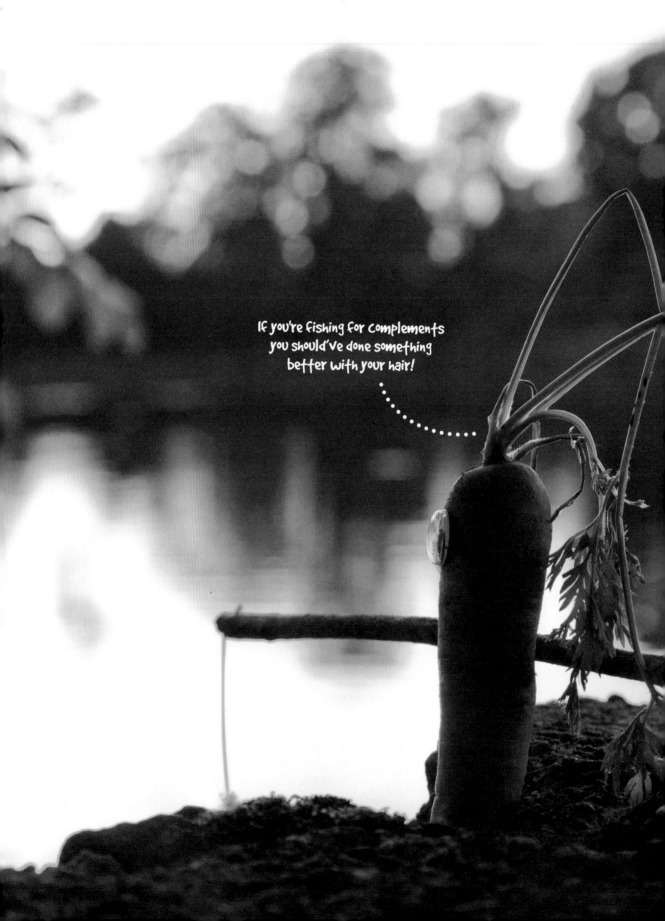

Contents

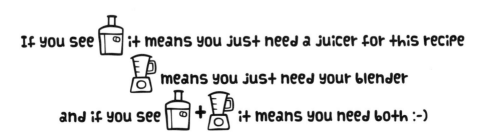

If you see 🧴 it means you just need a juicer for this recipe
🧃 means you just need your blender
and if you see 🧴 + 🧃 it means you need both :-)

Thank You!

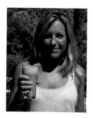

This is Katie, my rock. It is impossible to convey in words my gratitude for all that you do. You have helped so much in the creation of this book and supplied some of the gorgeous recipes and supported me every step of the way on my journey to *Juice The World*. **THANK YOU**. You complete me (now someone get the bucket! :-)) I would also like to congratulate you on taking the picture that made the inside front cover – these days it's just point and shoot!! ;-)

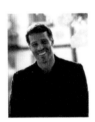

Hey, Tony Robbins! What can I say – "You're my ambassador of Kwan man" (or Quan, no one really knows how to spell it!). Thank you for all you do. You changed my life many years ago and helped to lift me from where I was then to where I am today. You are without question the world's number one. **THANK YOU** for helping to change the world in so many ways. By the time you have read this we should have already done lunch in Palm Springs (thanks for the invite!)

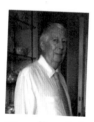

This is Lord Phil Harris of Peckham. Thank you for the contribution to the book and congratulations on losing 3 stone (42 lbs) in 3 months after reading the *7lbs in 7 days Super Juice Diet*, as well as bringing down your cholesterol by 3 points during that time. I'm a "Peckham boy" too and on behalf of all the people you help in South-East London particularly, I'd like to say a massive **THANK YOU**.

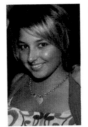

This is Robyn, my beautiful goddaughter, who never ceases to surprise and amuse me. She has nothing to do with this book or the Juice Master business but I love her and want to **THANK HER** for continually bringing sunshine into my world.

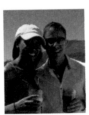

This is the Beverley Knight. Thanks soul diva! Great recipe and I've told you a few times, but I will never forget when you got up with no music and sang at my retreat in Turkey. You blew everyone away. **THANK YOU** for helping to spread the juicy word and thank you for sharing your incredible voice with the world.

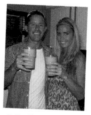

This is Katie Price, aka Jordan. You have done so much to help get so many juicing that I need to say a massive **THANK YOU**. Many people do not know the real Katie Price, but I personally think you are an incredible woman and more over, a truly extraordinary mother... if only people knew what really goes on hey. Thank you also for your recipe - nice!

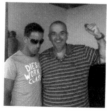

THANK YOU Phil Taylor for showing the world that not all Darts players survive on beer and chips! As you said - in order to keep at the very top of your game you need your body and mind to be sharp - thank you for helping to spread the juice revolution!

And Thank You To Everyone Who Has Helped In Some Way

You know who you are, and sorry I ran out of space – love you all x

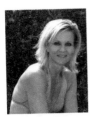

Hey **Linda Barker**, **THANK YOU** for the recipe baby. I was surprised to see you didn't insist on it being served in a glass covered in red velvet, but then I remembered that's Laurence Llewelyn-Bowen's style, not yours!

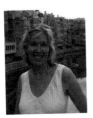

Without **Wanda Whitely**, my first book would never have been published. Wanda worked at Harper Collins at the time my manuscript landed on her desk. She read four chapters, called me up and said, "It's the best thing I have read on the subject of diet and health in 25 years". By the end of that week she had signed me up and the rest is history. **THANK YOU** Wanda, you will never be forgotten.

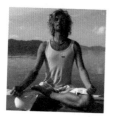

THANK YOU to the beautiful soul that is **Kenny Ryan**, the man who lives in a cave and is way beyond a 'yoga teacher'. You have been spreading your unique blend of Kenny magic since my very first health retreat and continue to do so today. **THANKS AN** and see you somewhere beautiful soon!

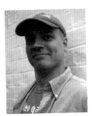

The Design King Of The World! The person who has put the "Funky" into this Funky Fresh Juice Book is **Alex Leith**. What can I say - you are "da man". **THANK YOU** dude and well done for hitting the deadline… time to sleep!

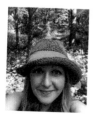

This is **Charlie**, wife of the Design King Alex and now a regular part of the juicy team. **THANK YOU** for laying out the many, many, many pages and helping to get the community juicers into the book. You're a star!

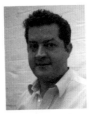

This is **John Pickering** (or JP as I like to call him). Juice Master's Ops Manager, and despite not being very good at table tennis, he's a pretty good Ops Manager. Moreover, I would like to **THANK YOU** for caring so much about what we do and for doing what it takes to help spread the juicy word to a global audience.

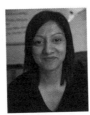

This is **Nina**, she's our retreats manager and probably the sweetest and most caring person you will ever meet. At first you may not see her, she is tiny! What she hasn't got in height (which is rich coming from little legs Vale!) she makes up for in heart. **THANK YOU** Nina, you have been with the company the longest and I'll never let you go, we all adore and love you very much :-)

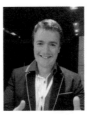

This is **David** (he is French so pronounced *Da-Vid*) **Jeanson**. What can I say other than a massive THANK YOU! You were with Moulinex and saw what I had to offer and then head-hunted me when you went to Philips. You have done so much to help my mission to *Juice The World* and I will never, ever forget that. You are passionate about all you do and it was your passion for juicing which helped change juicing forever. **THANK YOU**!

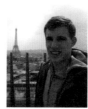

This is **Daniel**… the web wizard! He's a man who can produce an amazing website in a nano second. It's largely because of Dan we get to hold four Global Juice Reboots a year, look out for the next one and know that when you see the website for it - this is the man who made it happen! **THANK YOU**!

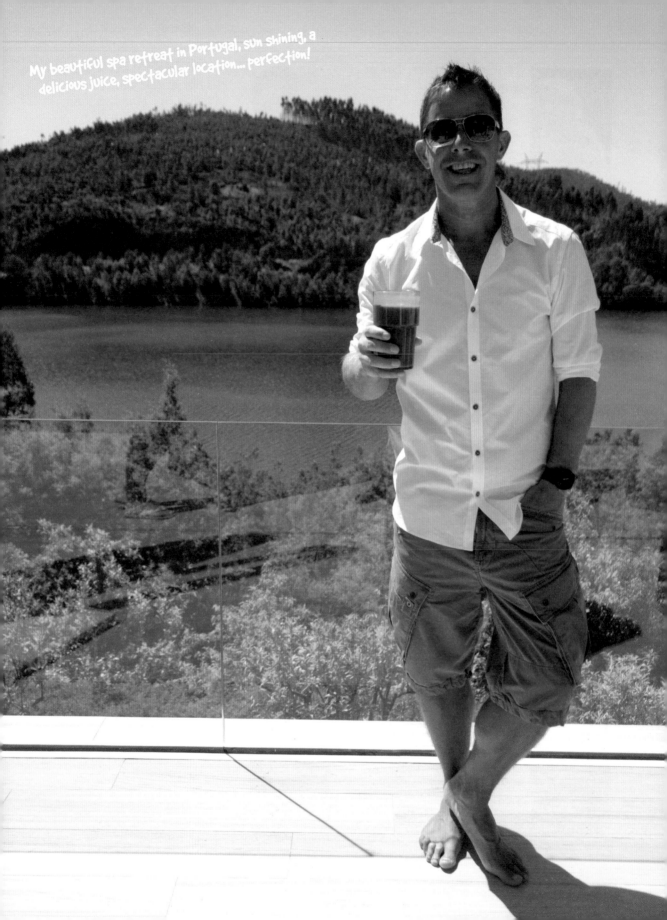

My beautiful spa retreat in Portugal, sun shining, a delicious juice, spectacular location... perfection!

The Juice Revolution

There is a revolution happening and I want you to be part of it! From **Bono** to *Simon Cowell*, from *Jennifer Aniston* to *Cheryl Cole*, fresh juicing is now becoming mainstream. More and more of us are opening our minds (and, of course, our mouths) to the incredible health benefits that freshly-extracted **live** juice has to offer.

Once the fad of a few Hollywood stars back in the late 70s and early 80s, fresh juicing is now becoming an important part of people's daily lifestyles. People are finally waking up to the importance of using nutrition for the treatment and – more importantly – the prevention of disease. People are beginning to understand that nature may just know a little more than even the most eminent scientists on earth when it comes to the precise nutritional elements required for optimum health. Many of us are starting to think with our own intuition, rather than simply buying what we are being fed daily by the pharmaceutical companies and corporations who have a vested interest in keeping us in fear and popping pills. We are starting to question the so-called "scientific studies" on medical drugs; we are looking into who conducted and funded those studies and who would be the main beneficiary of a positive outcome. And more and more of us are starting to realize that one of the best kept "secrets" to optimum health, mental sharpness and life-giving energy lie in the pure natural and organic liquid that flows within every single fruit and vegetable designed for human consumption. We are also starting to realize that if we really want to take full control of our own health and that of our families, then raw live nutrition must pass our lips *every single day*.

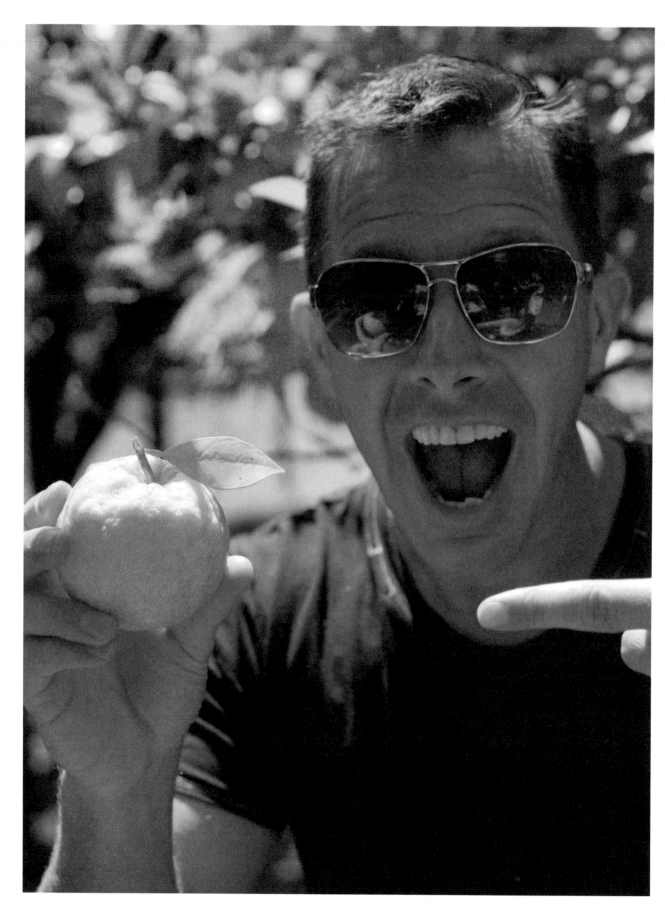

Let's Juice The World!

I have been writing and lecturing on the tremendous health benefits of freshly extracted juice for well over a decade. Every single day I hear of yet another story of how freshly extracted juice has totally transformed somebody's life.

When I first discovered the incredible power of this natural liquid fuel, I made it my "mission" to "Juice The World" – a goal that remains firmly at the centre of my life today. That mission has been totally cemented due to the health and life changes I have experienced myself, and seen in others, over the years.

It was my own ill health that led me on my journey of juicy discovery. I was covered from head to toe in a skin condition called psoriasis, to the point where almost every inch of my body – including my face – was affected. I was badly asthmatic, using an inhaler up to 14 times a day! I had extreme hay fever to the degree that I had to seek refuge in *any* air-conditioned building I could find. I was also overweight; a 40–to–60 a day smoker; and let's say I *liked* the drink.

When I started to pour this pure healing liquid inside my body I saw my own life and health drastically transform and I have witnessed tens of thousands of others do the same.

Nature's Liquid Pharmacy

What I refer to as "juicy communities" are popping up all over the world. People who have experienced such drastic changes to their mental and physical health that they want to tell as many people as they can to encourage others to a juicy life. This has created a ripple effect, and more and more people are starting to understand that a juicer is not simply a piece of kitchen equipment, but a catalyst to optimum mental and physical health. It's like having your own natural juice pharmacy on tap (or spout) whenever you like – no prescription or consultation needed.

With that in mind I created a "Dr Juice" section for this book, which contains specific juices that may help 15 of the most common ailments. Whether it's hay fever, asthma, arthritis, high cholesterol, diabetes, high blood pressure or psoriasis – nature usually has something up its nutritional sleeve that can help in some way.

Our Global Juicy Community

In the "Our Juicy Community" section of this book, you will also find a handful of juices and smoothies from a very small selection of our juicy "family". You will see they haven't *only* supplied their favourite recipe, they have also shared their amazing stories. You cannot read them and *not* feel totally inspired to get yourself and your family into a juicy way of life!

I have also added a "Kidz Corner" section with recipes from a few of the little ones in our juicy community. I think you may feel that a miracle has taken place when you start to see your little ones drinking vegetables like broccoli, carrot and spinach! And I have included a couple of tips at the start of that section to show how easy it is to get kids drinking vegetables – so make a point of reading it!

The Power of Juice

When you pour this perfect liquid fuel into your system daily it doesn't simply affect your general health – but every aspect of your life!

Beauty comes from within; and once you start to hydrate your body with the most carefully thought-out and "scientifically" put-together, nutritionally-perfect, organic liquid – everything shines! Your hair, your skin, your nails, your eyes, your thoughts, the whole **you**! When your body and mind start running on the fuel which was specifically designed by nature to flow through your blood – you feel fired up! This positively affects every single aspect of your life: your work, your business, your relationships, your confidence!

I cannot overstate what the right *live* fuel can do for you! It's like adding super-unleaded instead of diesel to an unleaded car. *Everything* you put into your body has an effect on your biochemistry. You know that even something simple like low blood sugar can affect your mood and energy. So imagine the effect that chucking dead rubbish into your bloodstream daily and the absence of optimum nutrition is having on your life. You will only really know just how much it affected your life when the right fuel starts to flow and your body starts running on what can only be described as "Super Fuel".

Juicing Is The New "Black"

I like to think I have had something to do with the juice "revolution" happening in many places around the world, today. My books on the subject have now sold over 2 million copies and have been translated into a variety of languages. My now infamous, *7lbs in 7 Days, Super Juice Diet* (known also as *The Juice Master Diet*) alone has sold over a million copies. It was an Amazon number 1 best-seller of all books, and even knocked the Da Vinci Code from the top spot on another book chart!

The message is spreading, and I will not stop until a juicer and blender becomes as common as a kettle and toaster in every house in the modern world. I honestly feel a juicer and blender is *that* important to modern life. It is, in my opinion, the best form of health insurance you and your family will ever own. It is certainly the tastiest health insurance on earth! Whilst we were always taught that "a spoonful of sugar helps the medicine go down", this *live* natural liquid "medicine" requires no "added anything" to help it go down. I understand that if you are new to fresh juicing you may feel that to get a vegetable juice down, you will indeed need some added sugar. However, I have been making vegetable based juices taste *divine* for over a decade; and even if you hate vegetables, you will **love** the recipes in this book!

No Added Salt
No Added Sugar
No Refined Fats
No Artificial Colours
No Artificial Flavourings
No Nasties What-so-ever!

The spectrum of vibrant colours you will see when making freshly extracted juice comes only from what nature provides. The creamy sweet delicious taste is sweetened simply by the natural sugars contained within the fruits and vegetables. The thick, rich texture and beautiful, slightly frothy head is the sign of pure "live" juice. You can be certain that when you make a fresh juice for you and your family, it will not only have no added anything, but it will also be…

100% Natural

100% Veggie

100% Raw

100% "Alive"

My aim for this book is a simple one. It's for you, your friends, and your family to join our juicy community and be part of **the Juice Master Revolution**. If you are already part of it, I hope this book will further cement your belief in fresh juice or re-ignite your juicy fire if it's started to fade at all.

Please make a point of reading the little "juicy facts" which accompany every juice and smoothie in this book. Some have good nutritional information and others are just quirky, random, funny facts designed simply to make you smile.

If you are brand new to juicing, make sure you read the "Funky, Fresh Juice Kitchen" (on the following pages) as you will need to know how to set up your very own juice bar at home. You will also need to know what juicer to get as there are some **very** bad ones out there, which could put you off juicing for life!

I will leave you to explore the book, indulge in some of the finest tasting nutrition on earth, and I sincerely hope you join our juicy revolution.

Please, spread the word, pass the book on, get a copy for your friends and the people you care about. You can even join us on Facebook 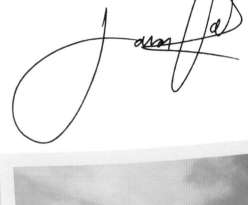 (just click "Like" on the Juice Master fan page) and also follow me on twitter @juicemaster.

Let's Juice The World Together!

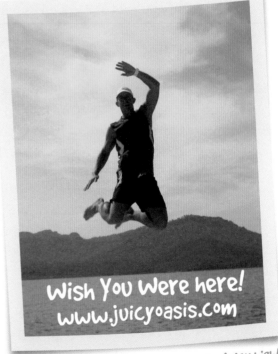

Wish you were here!
www.juicyoasis.com

No camera tricks – just on a genuine juicy high!

Your Funky Fresh Juice Kitchen

The Juicer

The first thing any funky, fresh juice kitchen needs is a great juicer. Juicing has come a long way since the nightmare juicers of the 1970s, 80s and even 90s. Back then, in order to make a fresh juice you needed to take a week off work and have the patience of Buddha. Okay so that's a *slight* exaggeration, but if you had a juicer back then – or you are living with a juicer from that time now – you will know that's not too far off the mark.

Juicers back then had very small feeding tubes, meaning that you had to spend an age cutting your fruit and veg into small pieces to fit them in. Then you had the problem of under-powered motors, which meant that the machine would virtually come to a stop when you pushed any hard fruit or veg in. The capacity to collect pulp was always tiny so you could only make juice for one or two people before having to stop and clean the machine. And that brings us onto the real bugbear of old juicers – the cleaning! They were so, **so, so** difficult and time-consuming to clean. In fact I would say the number one thing, which puts people off juicing, is the cleaning.

21st Century "Broadband" Juicing

The good news is juicing has caught up with the 21st century and juice extractors have gone "broadband", so to speak. The vast majority of juicers now come with a wide chute, which usually allows for 2 or 3 apples to be juiced whole – no chopping, no peeling, no hassle!

However, not all wide-funnel juicers are built the same. There are many coming in "off the shelf" from Asia, and big companies are simply adding their name to often inferior juicers. Many are very poorly made and many of them lack the ability to actually juice. Yes you *can* get juice from them, but often the pulp contains as much juice as the juice itself. When you buy a juice extractor you need a machine that does "exactly what it says on the tin" (so to speak), i.e. extract the juice efficiently from the fibres.

WHICH? Juicer

For years I have been recommending the *Philips Alu* juicer. WHICH? *Magazine* in the UK voted this juicer BEST BUY; *The Gadget Show* also had it as their best buy; it was called "the King Of Juicers" by Gadget Girl in another magazine; the Mirror newspaper gave it 10/10; and *Good Housekeeping Magazine* voted it BEST BUY too... and it's the one I recommend – at the time of writing this – above all others. Plus you get a FREE copy of one of my books with it, so you can pass it on to the people you love.

As I write this, *Philps* have just bought out a brand new juicer called *"The Avance"* and it's getting nothing but **5 star reviews**. They have completely turned juicing on its head with this model by flipping the filter mesh upside down. This drives the pulp into the base, which means you see beautiful juice as you make your concoctions and not messy pulp. With the pulp in the bottom, you simply lift out the tray and empty in the bin, making *The Avance* one of the easiest to clean juicers I have ever used.

The Avance may not be available in your country. It's not in the US, for example, but the *Jason Vale Fusion Juicer* is. Please always check the website to see what's hot in the juicing world. If you get the wrong juicer for your needs it can be an instant nail in your juicer coffin!

Masticating Juicers

If you are a juice connoisseur, you may notice that I haven't mentioned masticating juicers. The reason is because this book is about funky, fresh, and fast juicing. It's about getting the vast majority of people on the juicy road with no hassle. Masticating juicers are usually very expensive, hard to clean and it takes a long time to make a juice. The argument for them is that many believe they make a superior juice in terms of nutrition as the juice is extracted slowly, using less heat friction and more of the nutrition remains. And it is true when you make a juice it takes a great deal longer to separate with a masticating juicer. So if you have the time and the money, masticating may be the way to go for you.

If you are using this book with a masticating juicer, you will have to adjust the instructions accordingly as I have designed this book to be used in conjunction with a whole-fruit juicer, like the Philips. I would say for 90% of people who need to juice, the best centrifugal on the market is the one to get and if you ever feel the need for a masticating juicer once you understand more about juicing, look into it then.

The Blender

In order to make the plethora of delicious shakes in this book, you will need an *awesome* blender. You can pay anything up to £500 for a home blender and there are some amazing ones out there. A good blender is the difference between having bits of fruit or avocado in your teeth and a smooth smoothie. They are after all called "smoothies" not "crunchies"! Check my website for my latest recommendations.

If you don't have a lot to spend (and let's face it, not many people do) there are some great "standard" blenders on the market. If you have the Philips juicer, then simply for aesthetics you may want to get the Philips Alu blender as they look pretty good together.

Unlike juicers, there are *loads* of great blenders out there. You even have the option of getting a hand-blender. These are great not only for making smoothies, but also for soups and things like pesto. Again check out the website first and do a little research.

The Other Funky Stuff You'll Need

There are one or two other "essentials" that you will need for your funky fresh juice kitchen... check the next page to find out!

Degradable Pulp Bags

These are life savers in terms of reducing cleaning time. You simply place them into the pulp container, lift out after juicing and throw onto the compost to degrade. You can get these little beauties from us if you like and indeed other places.

Ice Trays

You'll probably have some already, but get some more. Not only will you be using a lot of ice, with recipes like the Juice Master's World-Famous Lemon … Aid (see p.53), you can freeze the juice into cubes and add to the next smoothie for speed.

Good Knives

Get yourself a decent fruit and veg knife and use it just for this job. A good knife is priceless at reducing the time spent making a juice.

Chopping Board

You probably have one already. I like wood, but it's your call. I also have a rather cool red one, which goes well with the fridge at Juicy HQ!

Kitchen Work Space

If you don't have room on your kitchen work-surface, as more and more appliances fight for prime space – make room! Nothing is more important than your juicer and blender, and your home juice bar should take priority over everything else, especially your microwave. Actually if you have a microwave and it's preventing you from setting up your juice station, pick it up and throw it through the window! No, but seriously… throw it at least in the bin. Also, once you have set up your juice station, never, **ever** show your juicer the cupboard… it will never see daylight again! Keep it out, primed and ready at all times.

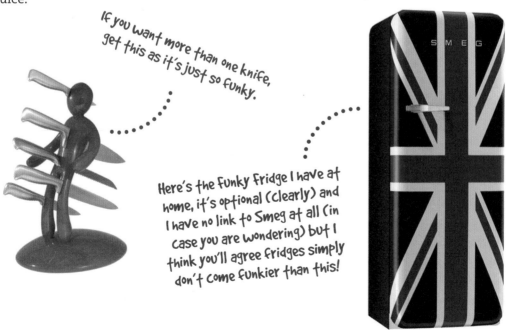

If you want more than one knife, get this as it's just so funky.

Here's the funky fridge I have at home, it's optional (clearly) and I have no link to Smeg at all (in case you are wondering) but I think you'll agree fridges simply don't come funkier than this!

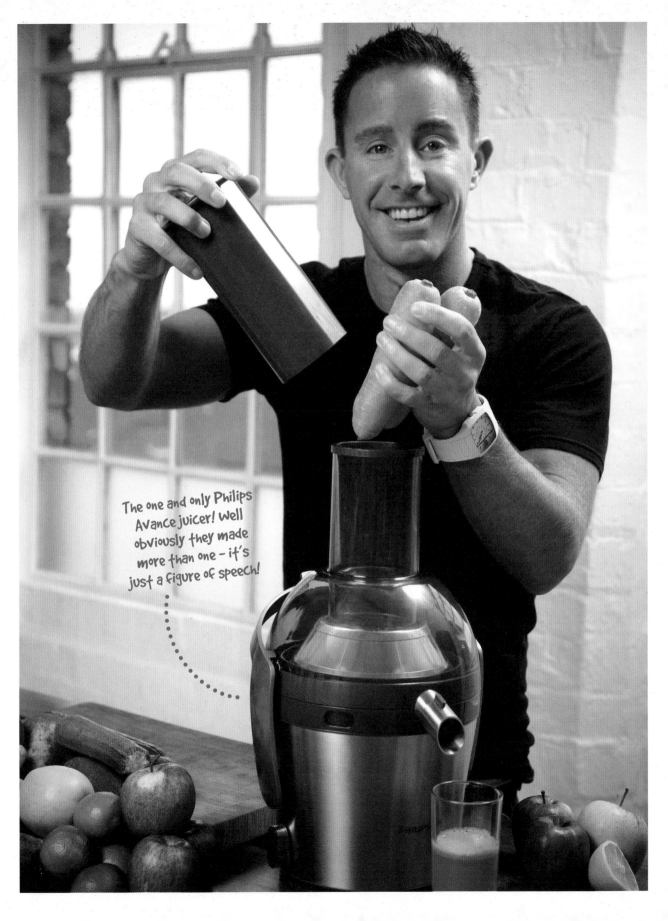

The one and only Philips Avance juicer! Well obviously they made more than one – it's just a figure of speech!

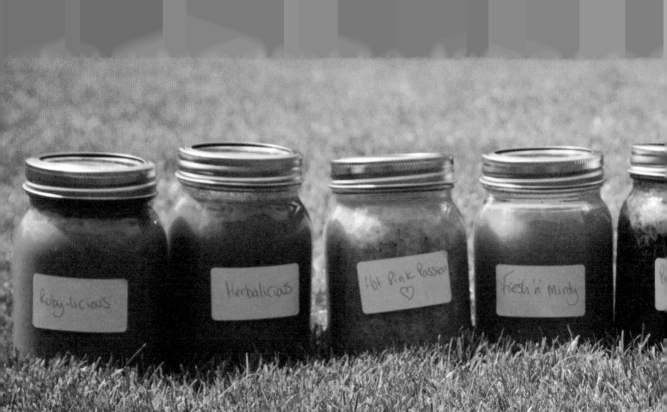

Juices & Smoothies

Unsure how best to describe the following selection of juices and smoothies? Here are some of the words others have used...

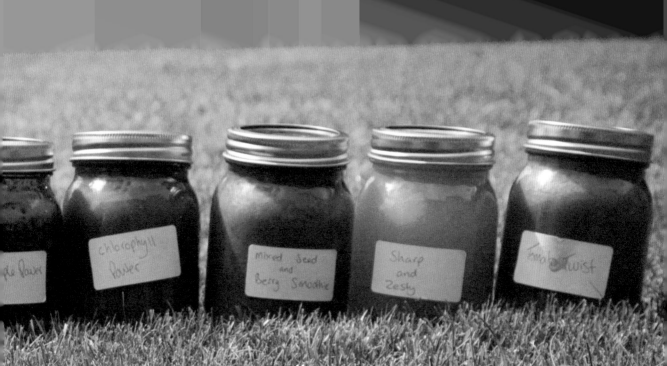

"oh so creamy"

"Nutritious and delicious"

"Mouth-watering"

"Scrummielicious"

"Beautifully indescribable..."

"wow!"

"A pure taste explosion"

"Divine"

"Yum! Yum! Yum!"

"Like droplets of heaven on your tongue"

"Sublime"

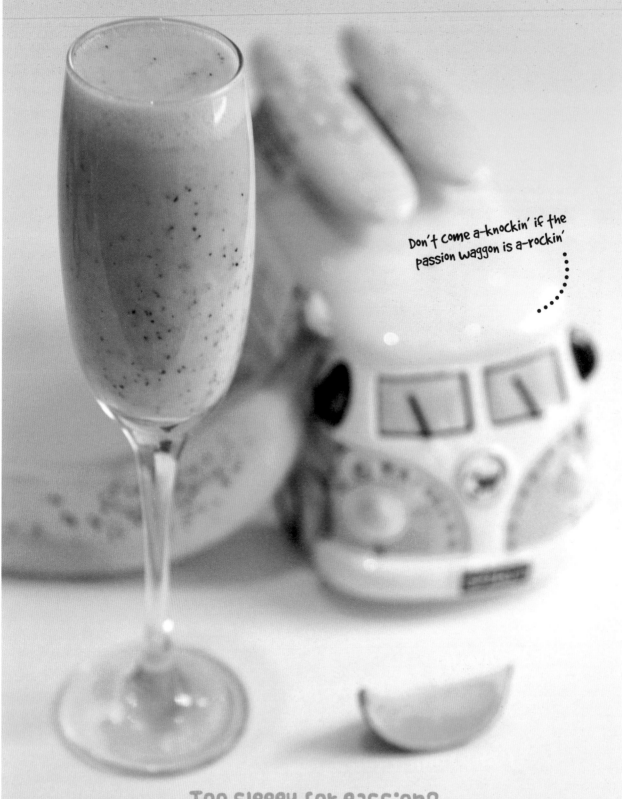

Too sleepy for passion?

Passion fruits are somniferous and when taken before bed can aid relaxation and restful sleep. So there may not be much passion, if you have any passion . . . fruit that is.

Passion, Pineapple, Banana & a Juicy Squeeze of Lime

Delicious freshly extracted pineapple juice, blended with a creamy banana, the flesh of two gorgeous passion fruit, a squeeze of lime and all cooled with some crushed ice.

Pineapple
1 medium

Lime
½ (peeled)

Banana
1 medium (ripe & peeled)

Passion Fruit
2 medium (peeled)

Ice
1 small handful

Let's Get Passionate

Peel the lime, leaving the white pith as it's where a great deal of the nutrients are to be found.

Juice the pineapple (no need to peel if you have a good juicer) and the lime.

Cut both the passion fruit in half, and scoop the flesh and seeds into the blender. Add the peeled banana, ice and the freshly extracted juice, and blend until delicious.

Best Served… in a frosted glass after a gorgeous passionate night with your partner… also loaded with zinc, which is essential for keeping things alive in *that* department!

Passionate About Passion Fruit

These tasty little fruits are rich in vitamin C and a good source of vitamin A, iron, and potassium. The seeds are also an excellent source of fibre. Passion fruit contains crunchy little seeds, which are edible. To eat them, cut in half and scoop out the insides with a teaspoon. Delicious and very good for you.

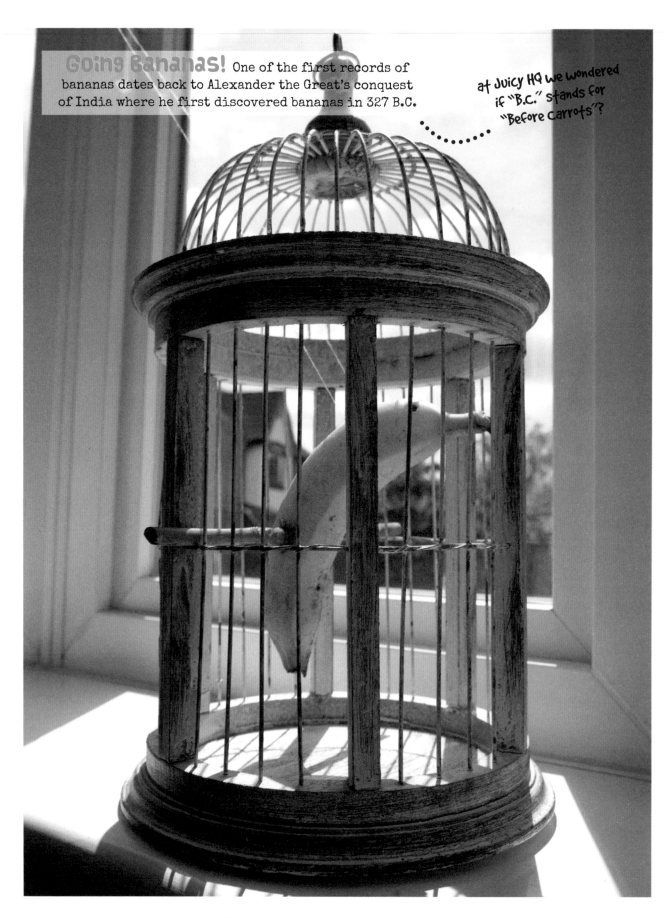

Going Bananas! One of the first records of bananas dates back to Alexander the Great's conquest of India where he first discovered bananas in 327 B.C.

at Juicy HQ we wondered if "B.C." stands for "Before Carrots"?

Pineapple, Banana, Cinnamon & Manuka Honey Shake

Every now and then at Juicy HQ we make certain combinations that just **send your taste buds into another galaxy** – this is one of those occasions!

Pineapple
½ medium

Banana
1 (ripe & peeled)

Manuka (Active) Honey
1 heaped teaspoon

Cinnamon
1 large pinch

Unsweetened Soya Milk
250 ml

Ice Cubes
1 small handful

A Little Glass Of Heaven

Juice the pineapple (no need to peel if you have a good juicer).

Put the peeled banana, Manuka honey, cinnamon, soya milk and ice into the blender. Add the fresh pineapple juice and blend until creamy.

Best Served... sitting on a FatBoy bean bag out in the sun in a cool and funky glass – the drink in the glass, not you, clearly!

Be Careful When Making This Smoothie!

In 2001, there were more than 300 banana-related accidents in Britain, mostly involving people slipping on skins!

You have been warned!

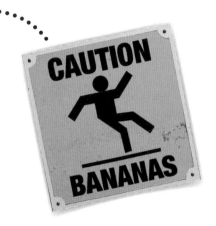

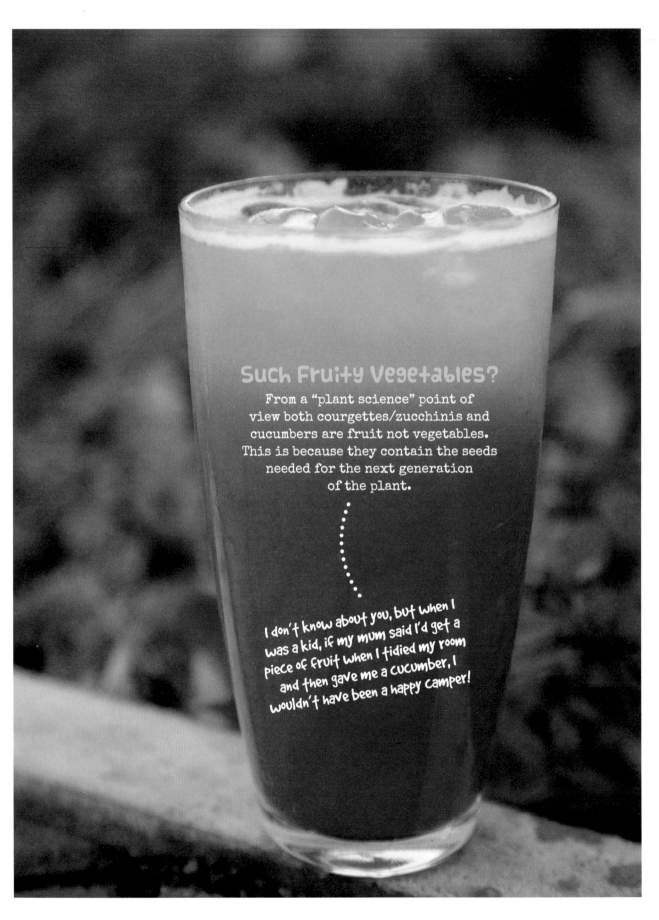

Such Fruity Vegetables?

From a "plant science" point of view both courgettes/zucchinis and cucumbers are fruit not vegetables. This is because they contain the seeds needed for the next generation of the plant.

I don't know about you, but when I was a kid, if my mum said I'd get a piece of fruit when I tidied my room and then gave me a cucumber, I wouldn't have been a happy camper!

Sooo Cool 'n' Sooo Zingy

Cool freshly extracted cucumber juice, creamy live apple juice, the thick texture of courgette juice, the bite of celery all "zinged" up with fresh ginger, zesty lemon and the unique aniseed flavour of fennel.

Sooo cool, sooo zingy, **sooo make it asap**!

Courgette / Zucchini
2 cm chunk

Fresh Ginger Root
1 cm chunk

Cucumber
¼ medium

Unwaxed Lemon
¼ (peeled)

Celery
½ stalk

Fennel
2 cm chunk

Golden Delicious Apples
2

Ice Cubes
1 small handful

How To Create This Juice

Peel the lemon, leaving as much of the white pith as possible to make the juice more nutritious.

Take the raw ingredients and then juice the lot!

Either pour the juice into a glass over ice or for a cooler juice, pop the lot in the blender with the ice and whizz to perfection.

Best Served...
from a glass because if you pour it straight into your hands it just makes a mess. Seriously though, it's a great juice when you want to cool down or fancy something a little zingy.

Rich In Vitamins & Minerals

Courgettes/zucchinis and cucumbers are a very good source of potassium, manganese, magnesium, vitamins A, C, K and folate. Both of these ingredients are wonderful for juicing as they have very mellow flavours and are a great base for a juice.

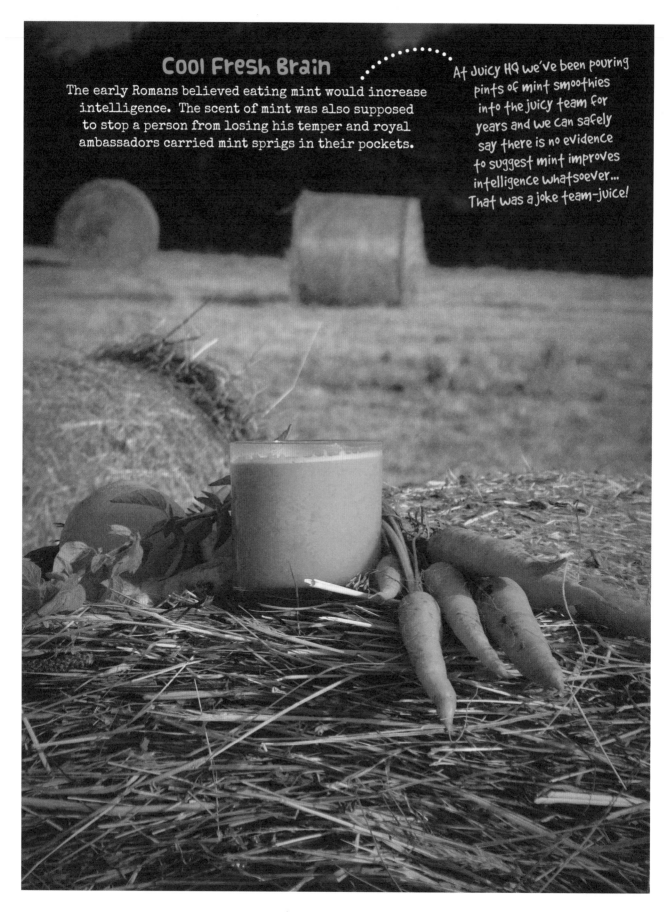

Cool Fresh Brain

The early Romans believed eating mint would increase intelligence. The scent of mint was also supposed to stop a person from losing his temper and royal ambassadors carried mint sprigs in their pockets.

At Juicy HQ we've been pouring pints of mint smoothies into the juicy team for years and we can safely say there is no evidence to suggest mint improves intelligence whatsoever... That was a joke team-juice!

Orange, Carrot, Mint 'n' Ginger

A taste sensation, a great combination:

A fruit, a vegetable, a herb and a spice,
This juice – it tastes **extremely nice**!

Juicy Oranges
2 (peeled)

Dark Carrots
2 medium

Fresh Ginger Root
½ cm chunk

Fresh Mint
1 handful

Ice Cubes
1 small handful

How To Make

This recipe works best with the juiciest oranges and darkest carrots you can find. Darker carrots contain more carotene, and juicier oranges are – well – juicier!

Peel the oranges, remembering to leave the white pith on to make the juice more nutritious.

Juice the oranges with the carrots and ginger.

Add the mint, ice and fresh juice to the blender. Whizz for 30 seconds, pour and enjoy.

Best Served... relaxing in a comfy hammock, watching the sun go down, but we at Juice Master HQ understand that a stool at your kitchen table may have to do.

So Good For You

Loaded with Beta Carotene, vitamins B, C, D, E and K, Minerals calcium, phosphorous, Potassium, Sodium

Posh Carrots

During the reign of Elizabeth I, the carrot became popular in England as a food and as a fashion accessory. Posh ladies would use carrot tops to decorate their hats. Well, we don't know about wearing them, but they certainly are a favourite in juices here at Juicy HQ!

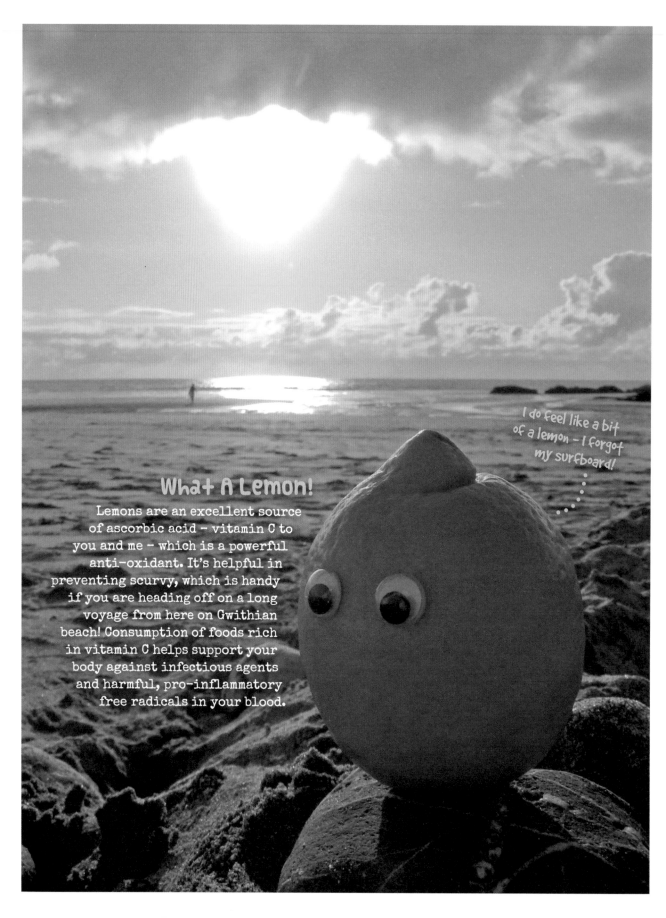

What A Lemon!

Lemons are an excellent source of ascorbic acid – vitamin C to you and me – which is a powerful anti-oxidant. It's helpful in preventing scurvy, which is handy if you are heading off on a long voyage from here on Gwithian beach! Consumption of foods rich in vitamin C helps support your body against infectious agents and harmful, pro-inflammatory free radicals in your blood.

I do feel like a bit of a lemon – I forgot my surfboard!

Cornish Lemon Surf

This **gorgeous lemon smoothie** was created just for this picture! I was in Cornwall while writing this book. I happened to have a juicy little lemon with me on the beach one evening and took this pic – it just had to go in the book! There's even a surfer in the background.

And **yes**, I do realize the name of this smoothie sounds like a laundry soap powder – thankfully it doesn't taste like one!

Unwaxed Lemon
1 (Cornish if possible)

Pineapple
⅓ medium

Bio-Live Yogurt
200 ml

Ice Cubes
1 small handful

Meet A Cornish Beauty

I realize that most lemon recipes bang on about Sicilian lemons – but let's keep it British with a nice juicy Cornish lemon! Clearly any lemon will do.

With a lemon zest grater, zest a small amount of the lemon peel and leave to one side.

Juice the pineapple (no need to peel if you have a good juicer) and the lemon (with the rest of the skin left on).

Pour the juice into the blender with the yogurt (if you are a vegan then you will need some soya yogurt) and ice, and blend until smooth.

Pour into a nice glass and sprinkle the lemon zest on top.

Best Served... sitting on a surfboard on Gwithian beach in Cornwall of course! Or close your eyes and drift there as you slowly sip this delicious "lemon curd" tasting smoothie... Yep! It actually *tastes like lemon curd!*

Why Bio-Live?

We use bio-live yogurt as it contains millions of friendly "helpers" which makes the lactose easier to digest, and supports the "good" bacteria in your digestive system. Plus it tastes better!

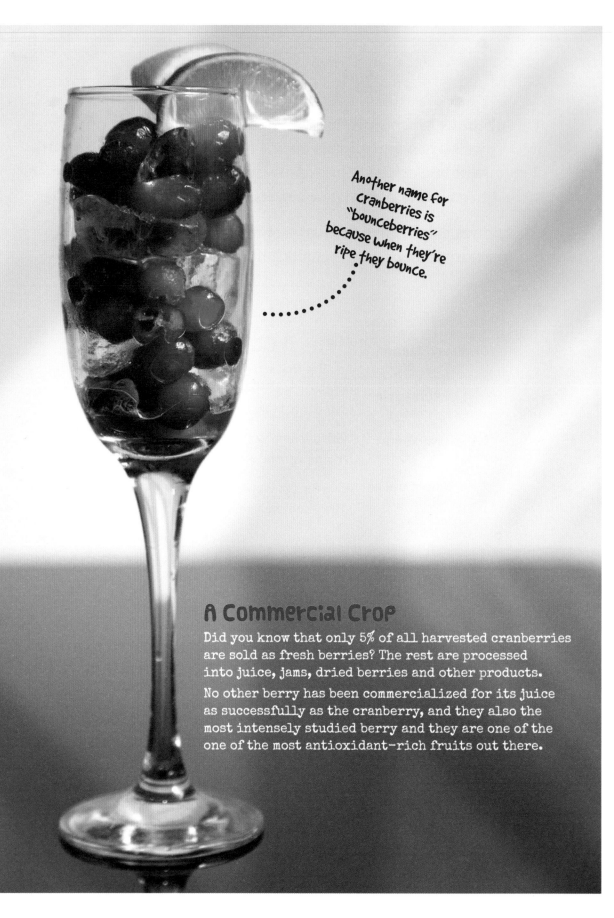

Another name for cranberries is "bounceberries" because when they're ripe they bounce.

A Commercial Crop

Did you know that only 5% of all harvested cranberries are sold as fresh berries? The rest are processed into juice, jams, dried berries and other products.

No other berry has been commercialized for its juice as successfully as the cranberry, and they also the most intensely studied berry and they are one of the one of the most antioxidant-rich fruits out there.

Cranberry Cosmo

A healthy twist on the timeless classic "The Cosmopolitan" made popular in recent times by Carrie Bradshaw in "Sex in the City". This juice is made from sweet, juicy oranges, sharp tart cranberries and zingy limes.

Indulge in this **little glass of sophistication**, safe in the knowledge that you wont be suffering with a sore head in the morning.

Oranges
2 (peeled)

Lime
½ (peeled)

Golden Delicious Apple
1

Cranberries
1 handful (fresh or frozen)

Ice Cubes
1 small handful

Be A Little Bit Cosmopolitan

Peel the oranges and lime, leaving as much of the nutrient-rich white pith as possible.

Juice the oranges, lime and apple.

Add the cranberries and ice to the blender, pour in the juice and blend. Remember that if you use frozen cranberries then there is really no need to add extra ice.

Best Served... in New York at some trendy rooftop bar — watching the city folk in their high-powered suits talking about Dow Jones, whoever he may be!

crantastic!

Cranberry juice is well known for its beneficial effect on urinary-tract infections and preventing cystitis in women. The juice helps to prevent bacteria from sticking to cell walls.

Cranberries are also abundant in flavonoids such as proanthocyanidins, flavonols and quercetin which have been found to have cancer-fighting properties.

Studies have even found that cranberry juice can prevent the formation of plaque on your teeth!

Now, if juice from a carton can do this, imagine the benefits of fresh "live" cranberry juice!

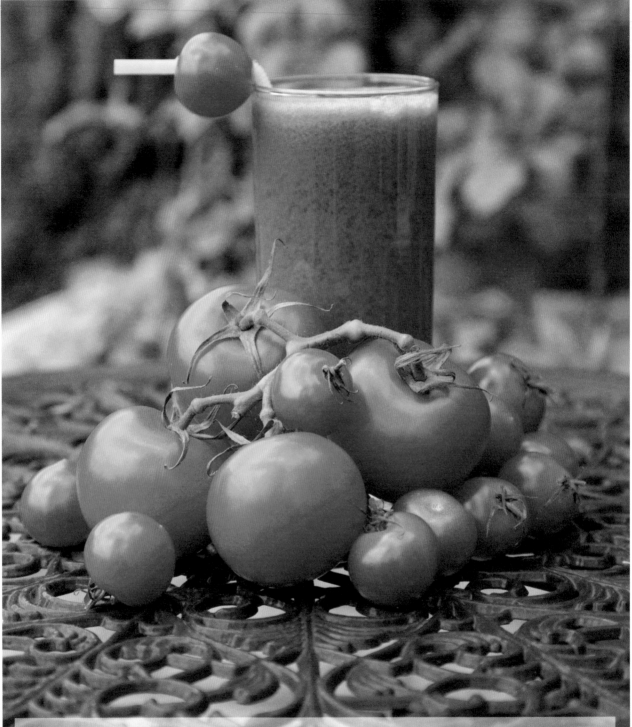

Made For Each Other!

American researchers have found that a combination of broccoli and tomato together is far more effective at reducing tumour growth in rats than individually. Tomatoes are rich in a powerful antioxidant phytochemical called lycopene that can protect the skin from sun damage and help to reduce inflammation in the body. Polyphenols in broccoli are thought to impair the growth of prostrate cancer cells.

Tomato Broccoli Twist

Pure tomato juice can be too thick and heavy. However adding a little water-rich broccoli, cucumber and celery juice, and lifting it with twist of lemon, creates a drink that's **in a different league on both the taste and nutrition front** to the traditional "tomato juice in a can".

"On The Vine" Tomatoes
3 medium

Broccoli
2 cm chunk

Cucumber
½ medium

Celery
1 stalk

Unwaxed Lemon
⅓

Ice Cubes
1 small handful

Let's Do The Twist

Pack the tomatoes (with the vines removed) tightly into the chute of the juicer and juice on the slowest speed, to extract the most juice. Juice the remaining ingredients.

Either blend with, or pour over, ice.

Best Served... on an empty stomach or if you fancy something more veg and less fruit. This is also a really great juice to serve to someone in hospital and much tastier and healthier than any hospital food.

When is a Fruit Not a Fruit?

Although technically tomato is a fruit it's rarely treated as one. Have you ever seen a fruit bowl with apples, oranges, bananas and tomatoes? The reason the tomato is a fruit is because it contains seeds which vegetables do not. So that means other veg that are actually fruit include bell peppers and cucumbers as well!

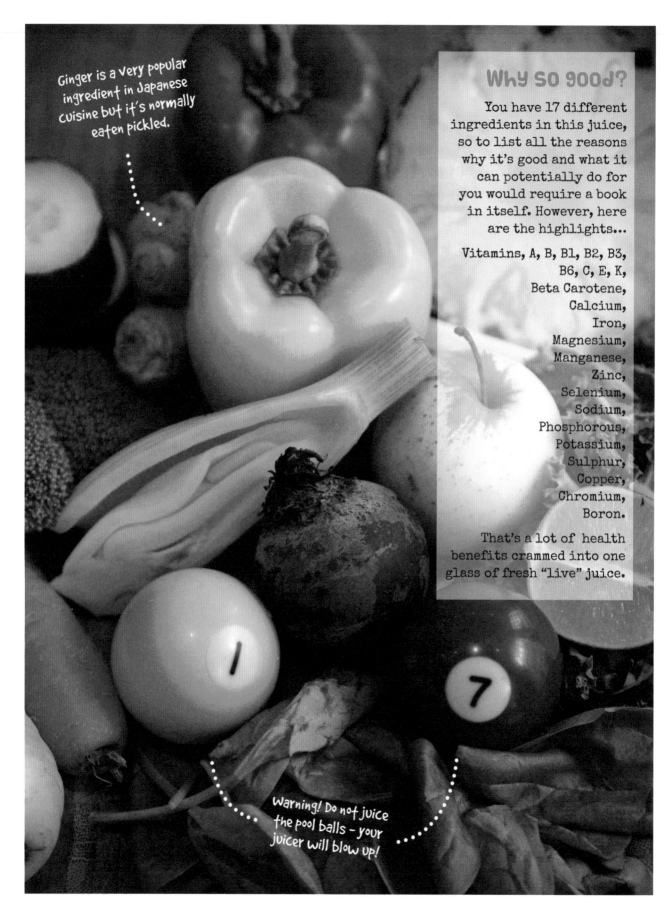

Ginger is a very popular ingredient in Japanese cuisine but it's normally eaten pickled.

Why so good?

You have 17 different ingredients in this juice, so to list all the reasons why it's good and what it can potentially do for you would require a book in itself. However, here are the highlights...

Vitamins, A, B, B1, B2, B3, B6, C, E, K, Beta Carotene, Calcium, Iron, Magnesium, Manganese, Zinc, Selenium, Sodium, Phosphorous, Potassium, Sulphur, Copper, Chromium, Boron.

That's a lot of health benefits crammed into one glass of fresh "live" juice.

Warning! Do not juice the pool balls – your juicer will blow up!

Japanese 17-a-Day

Did you know that Japanese RDA (recommended daily allowance) of fruits and vegetables is **17 different portions**, yet most governments recommend we consume just five? With Japan being home to some of the planet's oldest living people, I'm more inclined to trust their recommendations than ours...

Golden Delicious Apple
1

Pear
1

Cucumber
2 cm chunk

Unwaxed Lime
½ small

Fresh Ginger Root
1 cm chunk

Spinach
1 small handful

Celery
½ stalk

Carrot
½ medium

Kale
1 small handful

Raw Beetroot
½ small

Pineapple
1 cm slice (peeled)

Broccoli Stem
1 cm chunk

Courgette / Zucchini
1 cm small

Parsnip
1 cm chunk

Fennel
1 cm chunk

Red Bell Pepper
1 small slice

Yellow Bell Pepper
1 small slice

Ice Cubes
1 small handful

That's "Hello Health" in Japanese

Say "Konichiwa Kenkou"

There may be 17 ingredients but this is surprisingly easy to make. Pack the leafy vegetables tightly into the chute of the juicer, between the apple and the pear, to ensure you extract the maximum amount of juice. Then simply juice everything else and pour over the ice.

Best Served... when you really feel you need a
massive boost of nutrients. Maybe you've just been on a bender and feel like you've been run over by a truck. Perhaps you have just eaten your weight in sugar and need some goodness. Whatever the reason, just get this amazing juice inside you.

Looking and Feeling Great!

Just the vitamin A alone found in this juice is important for vision, growth, bone-building, the reproductive system and the mucus membranes. Vitamin A also helps to nourish skin, teeth and gums. That's before we get onto anything else!

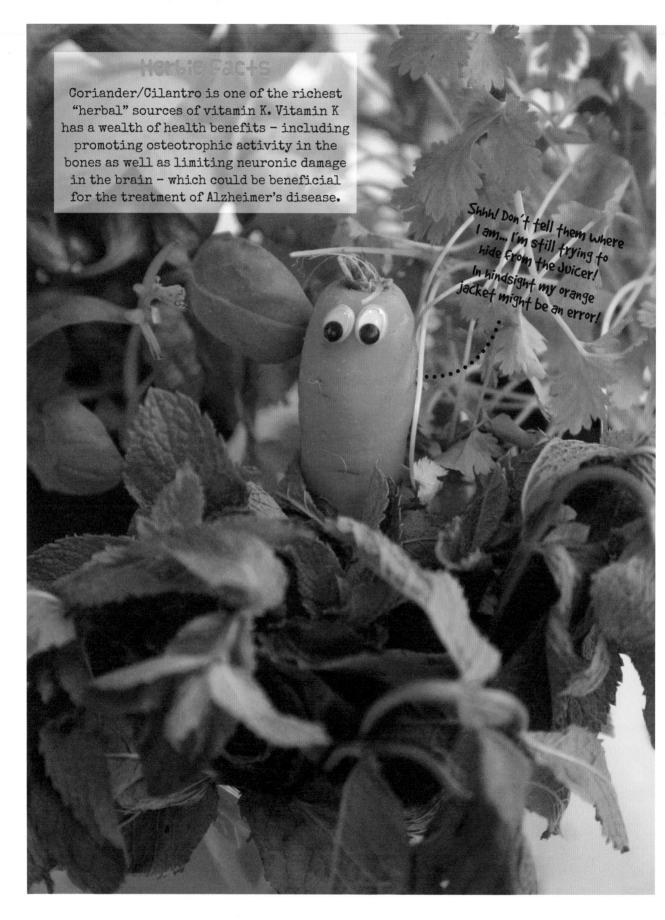

Herbalicious!

I'm not a herbalist, but I am aware of just how powerful herbs can be. This combination of every-day herbs is really **quite wonderful on the taste front**. Moreover, it's **extremely powerful on the health front** too.

"Bug" as in "Herbie", you know:
VW "Bug"… oh never mind!

Golden Delicious Apples
2

Carrots
2 medium

Fresh Coriander / Cilantro
leaves of 4 sprigs

Fresh Basil
leaves of 4 sprigs

Fresh Mint
leaves of 4 sprigs

Lime
½ (peeled)

Ice Cubes
1 small handful

Get The "Bug" For This Smoothie

Peel the lime, leaving behind as much of the white pith as you can.

Juice the apples, carrots and lime. Make sure you sandwich the lime between the apples to get the most juice.

Pour the juice into a blender, add the herbs, ice and blend.

Best Served… sitting under a gorgeous tree in the herb garden at the spectacular Cowley Manor near Cheltenham in rural England. If you ever stay there and ask them to make this juice, they will oblige – as nothing seems to be too much trouble. Maybe once you're finished you can relax at their outside pool…

Mineral Rich Herbs

Coriander/Cilantro is a good source of minerals like potassium, calcium, manganese, iron, and magnesium. Potassium in an important component of cell and body fluids that helps control heart rate and blood pressure. Iron is essential for red blood cell production. And manganese is an essential nutrient used by many enzymes in the brain and body.

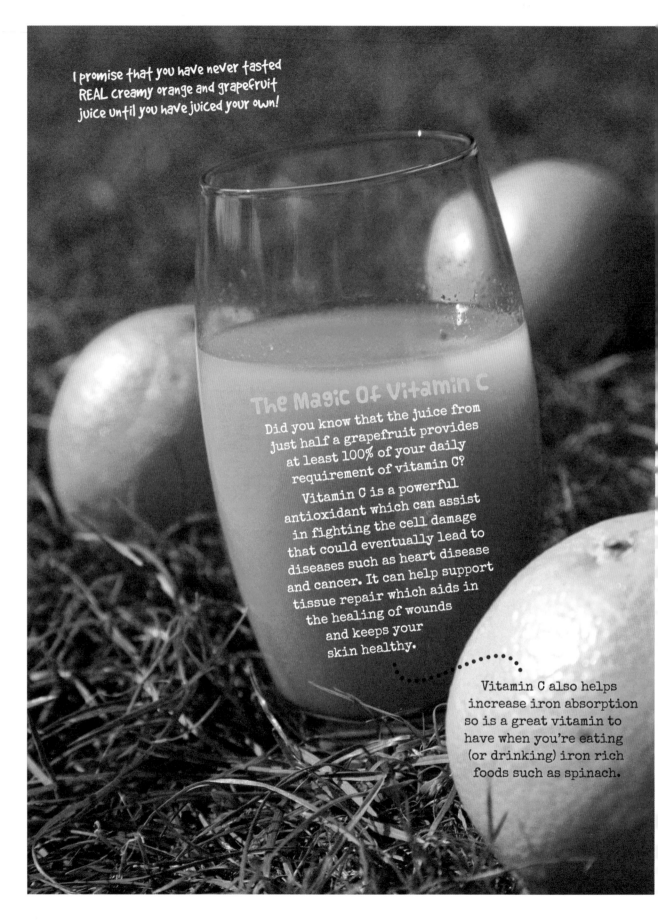

I promise that you have never tasted REAL creamy orange and grapefruit juice until you have juiced your own!

The Magic Of Vitamin C

Did you know that the juice from just half a grapefruit provides at least 100% of your daily requirement of vitamin C?

Vitamin C is a powerful antioxidant which can assist in fighting the cell damage that could eventually lead to diseases such as heart disease and cancer. It can help support tissue repair which aids in the healing of wounds and keeps your skin healthy.

Vitamin C also helps increase iron absorption so is a great vitamin to have when you're eating (or drinking) iron rich foods such as spinach.

A Taste Of Florida

Palm Beach, Miami, The Keys, Clear Water, Tampa Bay… the list of beautiful places in Florida just goes on and on. The "Sunshine State" is also well know for producing some of the **most gorgeous oranges and grapefruits in the world**. Luckily, you don't have to hop on a plane to get hold of them as Florida oranges and grapefruits can be found on this side of the pond for most of the year.

It will come as no surprise that this "Taste Of Florida" juice has a combination of freshly extracted Florida orange and pink grapefruit, with a touch of lime.

Florida Oranges
3 medium (peeled)

Florida Pink Grapefruit
½ medium (peeled)

Lime
1 small (peeled)

Ice Cubes
1 small handful

How To Get Florida In A Glass

Clearly, if you can't get hold of *Florida* oranges and *pink* grapefruit you can, of course, use other varieties.

Peel the oranges, grapefruit and lime, leaving as much of the white pith as possible.

Juice the lot and pour over ice.

Best Served… in a cool glass on a deck chair perhaps (or a beach towel) watching the sunrise over Cocoa beach or the sunset over the White Sands!

Failing that why not put on your favourite beach tunes, close your eyes, take a sip and imagine yourself there.

Growing Up With Vitamin C

Vitamin C is important for body growth and is an essential vitamin for growing children. But did you also know that Vitamin C has been shown to dramatically reduce blood lead levels? This could be important for children growing up in urban areas as studies show that lead toxicity can lead to behavioural and developmental problems, such as learning disabilities and even lowered IQ.

Perhaps instead of milk they should be giving kids freshly extracted orange juice at school.

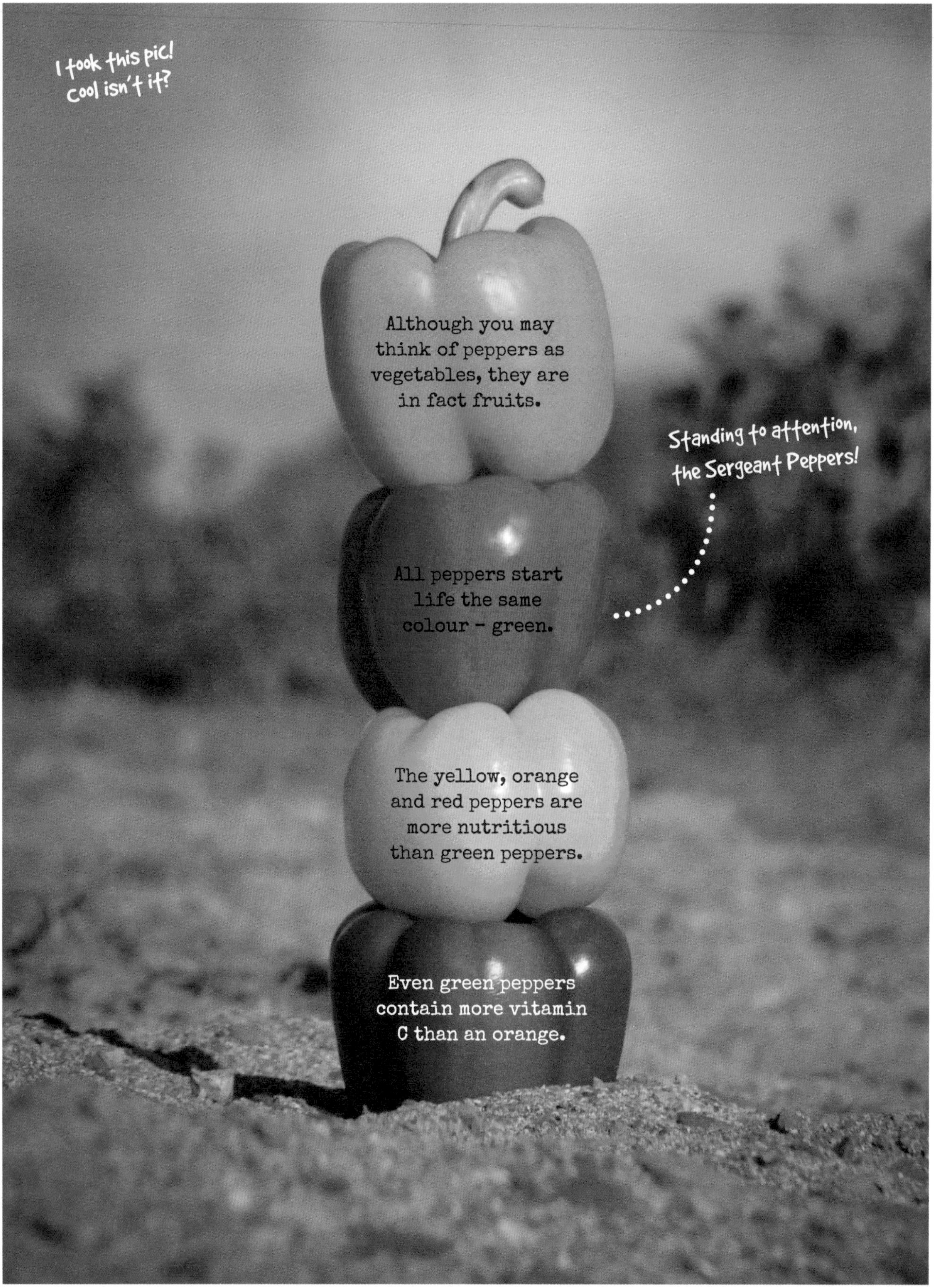
I took this pic! Cool isn't it?
Although you may think of peppers as vegetables, they are in fact fruits.
Standing to attention, the Sergeant Peppers!
All peppers start life the same colour - green.
The yellow, orange and red peppers are more nutritious than green peppers.
Even green peppers contain more vitamin C than an orange.

The Fab Four

The peppery one! Gorgeous, sweet – *yes*, I said "sweet" – nutrient rich, multi-coloured bell peppers, mixed with the creamy juice of pineapple and apple, and the cooling juice of cucumber. Don't knock it 'til you've tried it!

In fact, don't knock it at all, it took me ages to stack those peppers up like that!

Pineapple
¼ large

Golden Delicious Apple
1

Cucumber
2 cm chunk

Orange **Bell Pepper**
¼ medium

Red **Bell Pepper**
¼ medium

Yellow **Bell Pepper**
¼ medium

Green **Bell Pepper**
¼ medium

Ice Cubes
1 small handful

She Loves You Yeah, Yeah, Yeah!

Juice the peppers as they are (no need to seed or core them). Then juice the pineapple (no need to peel if you have a good juicer), apple and cucumber.

Pour into a lovely tall glass over the ice.

Best Served... on an empty stomach. Like nearly all of the recipes in this book, it is very filling, but will take about 15 minutes for your body to register. So don't eat anything at the same time, or you'll be stuffed... like a pepper!

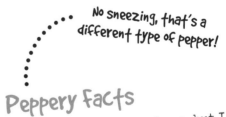

No sneezing, that's a different type of pepper!

Peppery Facts

Bell peppers are named after their shape, but I think they look more like Chinese lanterns.

Peppers stop ripening once picked, and the different colours are simply different stages of ripeness.

Peppers are loaded with silicon, which is great news for hair, nails and skin.

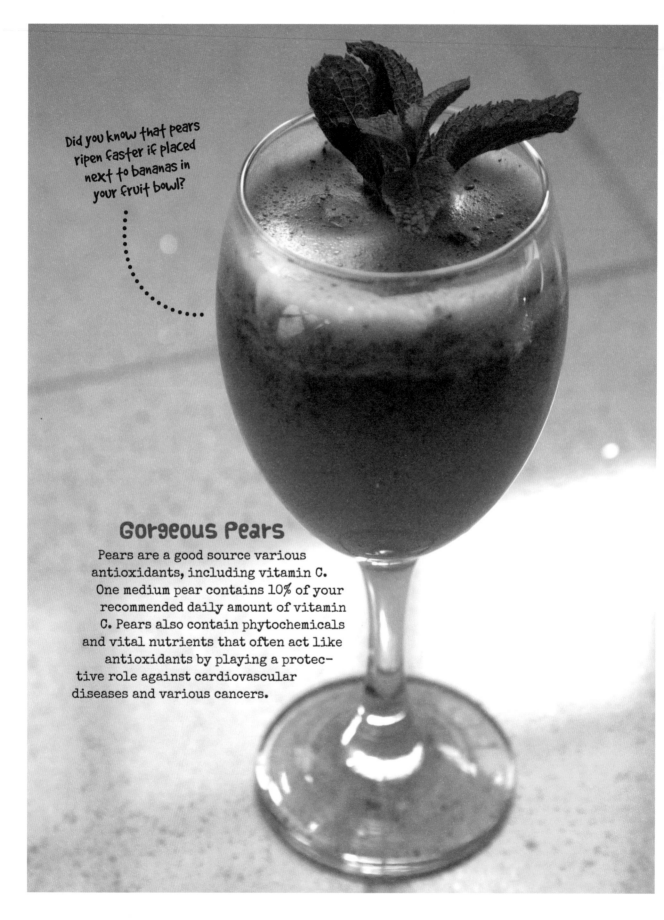

Did you know that pears ripen faster if placed next to bananas in your fruit bowl?

Gorgeous Pears

Pears are a good source various antioxidants, including vitamin C. One medium pear contains 10% of your recommended daily amount of vitamin C. Pears also contain phytochemicals and vital nutrients that often act like antioxidants by playing a protective role against cardiovascular diseases and various cancers.

Pear 'n' Mint Magic

The juice of fresh, thick pears and zesty lime blended with fresh mint. You've just created a unique juice harmony that is simply too good to describe – well OK I'll give it a go, how about "*magic*"?

Pears
2 medium

Cucumber
¼ medium

Lime
½ (peeled)

Fresh Mint
leaves of 4 sprigs

Ice Cubes
1 small handful

How To Create Magic

Peel the lime, leaving as much of the white pith as you possibly can.

Juice the pears, cucumber and lime by sandwiching the lime between the pears.

Pour the fresh juice into the blender. Add the leaves of mint and ice, and blend for a few seconds.

Best Served... "When you are stuck like Sticky the Stick Insect on a sticky bun" – a cool line straight from perhaps the best British comedy series in all of history – Black Adder. Apart from series one of course, which was just odd! To be honest, this juice should really have been called the "unblocker" and added to the Dr Juice section!

Keep on Going!

The oils in mint are very effective at relieving digestive discomfort. They're an antispasmodic and help to relax the muscles that line the walls of the intestines, breaking down and removing gas from the gut. The mint combined with the soluble fibre of the pear juice will almost be like a free colonic.

...umm, not sure if that might now put you off! Don't worry it's a great tasting juice!

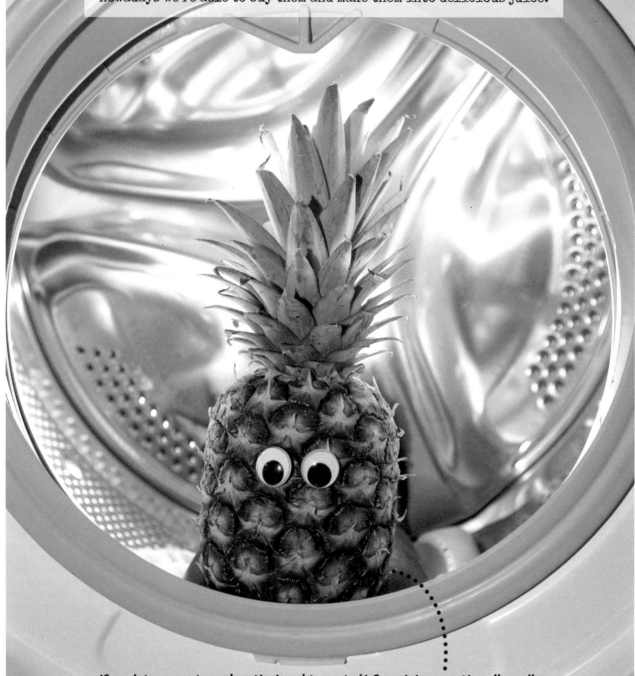

Posh Pineapples

When pineapples were first introduced to England during the reign of Charles II they were so rare that only the very rich could afford them. Also, they were also not eaten, they were used as a symbol of wealth – put on display and left to rot! Thank heavens nowadays we're able to buy them and make them into delicious juice.

If you juice your pineapple with the skin on, don't forget to wash it really well. Perhaps this is a bit over the top though!

Pineapple Colada

The virgin version of this Hawaiian favourite combines smooth and creamy coconut milk with the sweet taste of pineapple. Make it even more creamy and indulgent by adding half a potassium-rich banana – *yummy, scrummy*!

Satsuma or **Tangerine**
1 medium (peeled)

Pineapple
½ medium

Coconut Milk
200 ml

Banana
½ (ripe & peeled) – optional

Ice Cubes
1 small handful

How To Create The Colada

Peel the satsuma or tangerine, leaving as much of the white pith as possible for a more nutritious juice.

Juice the satsuma or tangerine with the pineapple (no need to peel if you have a good juicer).

Pour the fresh juice into the blender. Add the coconut milk, banana (if desired) and ice, and blend.

Best Served... under a palm tree in St Lucia. If you can't get there, then serve this delicious juice in a cool frosted glass as a replacement for lunch. It's great if you are looking to drop some weight as it's very filling and will keep you off the muffins for many hours!

Are you coconuts?!

Yes it's true, coconuts contain saturated fats, but not all fats are the same. The fat found in coconut is lauric acid, which is also found in mothers milk and has many nourishing properties. Lauric acid has anti carcinogenic, antimicrobial, antibacterial, and antiviral properties. This helps to fight off viruses, boost healthy brain development and is vital for strengthening bones.

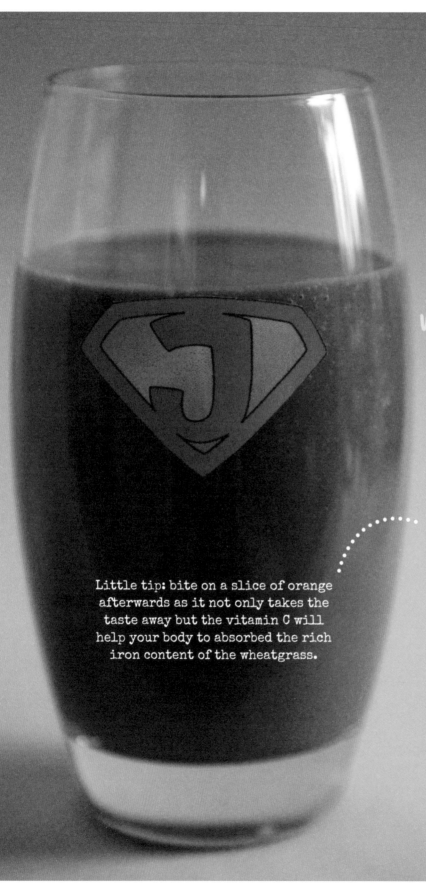

Wheatgrass Tips

Not everyone loves the strong taste of wheatgrass. If you don't like it we recommend that you don't add it to this juice; instead why not have the shot as a "chaser" and gulp it down in one go, trying not to pull a face of course!

Little tip: bite on a slice of orange afterwards as it not only takes the taste away but the vitamin C will help your body to absorbed the rich iron content of the wheatgrass.

If you are going to pull a face, please make sure it's yours as people tend to get offended when you pull their face! Just sayin'!

Juice Master's Green Super Smoothie

There has never been a better time to go green and if it's a **powerhouse of pure nutrients** you want, then this is the smoothie for you! Rich in chlorophyll, all the essential amino acids, essential fats, vitamins, minerals, and natural sugars – it's the daddy of green smoothies!

Golden Delicious Apples
2 medium

Spinach
1 large handful

Kale
1 large handful

Unwaxed Lime
½ small

Celery
1 stick

Cucumber
½ medium

Broccoli Stem
5 cm chunk

Avocado
½ medium

Spirulina
1 heaped teaspoon

Wheatgrass
1 fl oz shot

Ice Cubes
1 small handful

Is It A Bird, Is It A Plane?

Juice the apples, spinach, kale, lime, celery, cucumber and broccoli. Make sure you pack the leafy vegetables tightly into the chute of the juicer between the apples before you start to get the maximum juice.

Pour the fresh juice into the blender with the avocado, spirulina, wheatgrass and ice. Blend until very green and very smooth.

If you don't have fresh wheatgrass you can replace the wheatgrass shot with 1 heaped teaspoon of powdered wheatgrass. But the fresh stuff really is the best!

Best Served... in front of as many people as possible to show how ridiculously healthy you are. If you only have one of these a day, make sure people know about it!

Super Spirulina!

Spirulina is a true superfood, bursting at the seams with nutrients! It's rich in vitamins E and C, minerals, chlorophyll, essential fatty acids, and more beta carotene than any other food (by weight). Spirulina also has the highest protein content of any plant food!

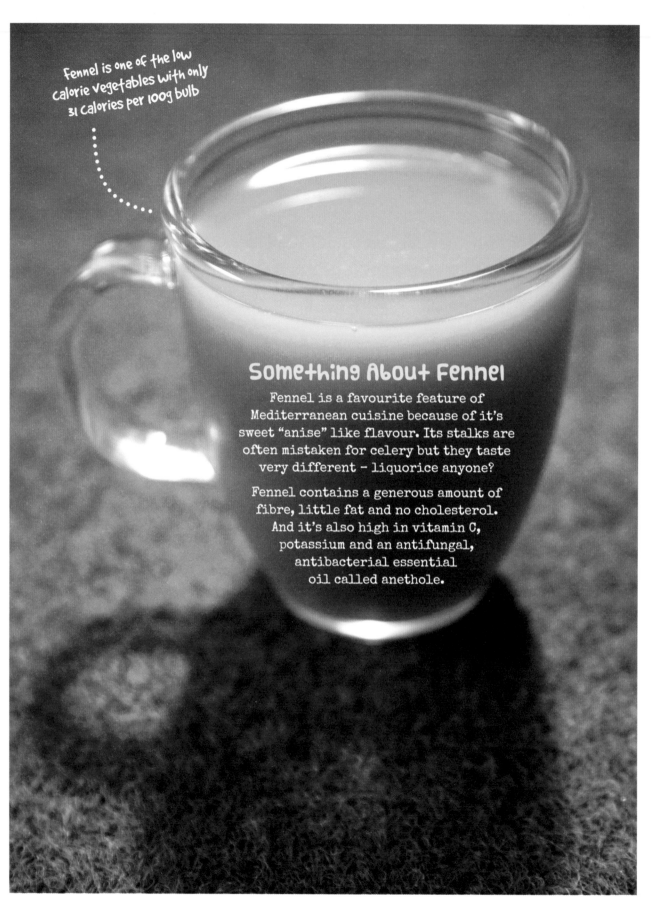

Fennel is one of the low calorie vegetables with only 31 calories per 100g bulb

Something About Fennel

Fennel is a favourite feature of Mediterranean cuisine because of it's sweet "anise" like flavour. Its stalks are often mistaken for celery but they taste very different – liquorice anyone?

Fennel contains a generous amount of fibre, little fat and no cholesterol. And it's also high in vitamin C, potassium and an antifungal, antibacterial essential oil called anethole.

Fennel, Spinach, Apple & Lime

If you didn't like those little aniseed ball sweets we all tried as kids – this may not be for you. However, if they were your idea of heaven then a juice that tastes very similar, but without the refined sugar and nasties, will be right up your street. A juice that **tastes like liquorice** – how lovely!

Golden Delicious Apples
2 medium

Fennel
1 bulb

Spinach
1 small handful

Lime
1 small (peeled)

Ice Cubes
1 small handful

How To Make

Peel the lime, leaving as much white pith as possible.

Juice the lot. Don't forget to pack the spinach tightly into the chute of the juicer, between the apples (before you turn the machine on), to get the most juice.

Pour over ice and enjoy.

Best Served... lying in the garden, sun beating down, phone off the hook (sorry – going back in time to when phones had a "hook" and we didn't have one permanently welded to our face!), radio on, reading a "junky" magazine to get the latest celeb gossip, knowing it's your day off and you have nothing else to do but relax. If that's dreamland, simply serve in a gorgeous glass, sip like a fine wine and just imagine yourself there.

Funky Fennel Facts!

Throughout history fennel has been revered as a medicinal herb. The Greek philosopher Hippocrates used it in medicine, and Romans believed that the young shoots could be eaten to control obesity. They were nearly right as the fennel seeds are known to be an appetite suppressant.

Fennel can also be helpful for indigestion and spasms of the digestive tract.

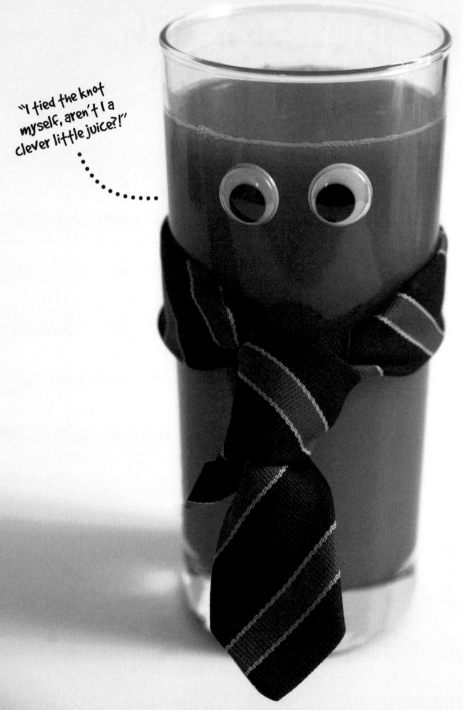

Why The School Shake Is Good For Little Brains

Students at a Twickenham school in the UK were recently helped through their exams by eating bananas at breakfast, break and lunch, in a bid to boost their brainpower. Researchers found that the potassium-packed banana can assist with learning by making pupils more alert. They're a great "fast food" as they regulate blood sugar and give a quick energy boost.

School Shake

The juiciest, freshest orange juice, mixed with the creamiest freshly extracted pineapple juice blended with sweet banana and ice.

Blood Oranges
2 medium (peeled)

Pineapple
¼ medium

Banana
1 large (ripe & peeled)

Ice Cubes
1 small handful

Shake It Up, Baby!

Peel the oranges, leaving the white pith to make the juice more nutritious and creamier.

Juice the pineapple (no need to peel if you have a good juicer) and oranges.

Pour the juice into the blender. Add the peeled banana and the ice, and blend until "too cool" smooth.

Best Served... in a mini flask, popped into their packed lunch. You'll have piece of mind knowing they're getting something nutritious at school, and they'll be none the wiser as it tastes too good to be good for you!

Also tell them "to shake well before drinking" – At least that way they'll be getting some exercise too!

Tip of The Banana

Why not peel your bananas from the bottom? Squeeze the black bit at the bottom, it will pop open and is much easier to peel. You won't have to pick the little "stringy bits" off of it either. That's how the primates do it.

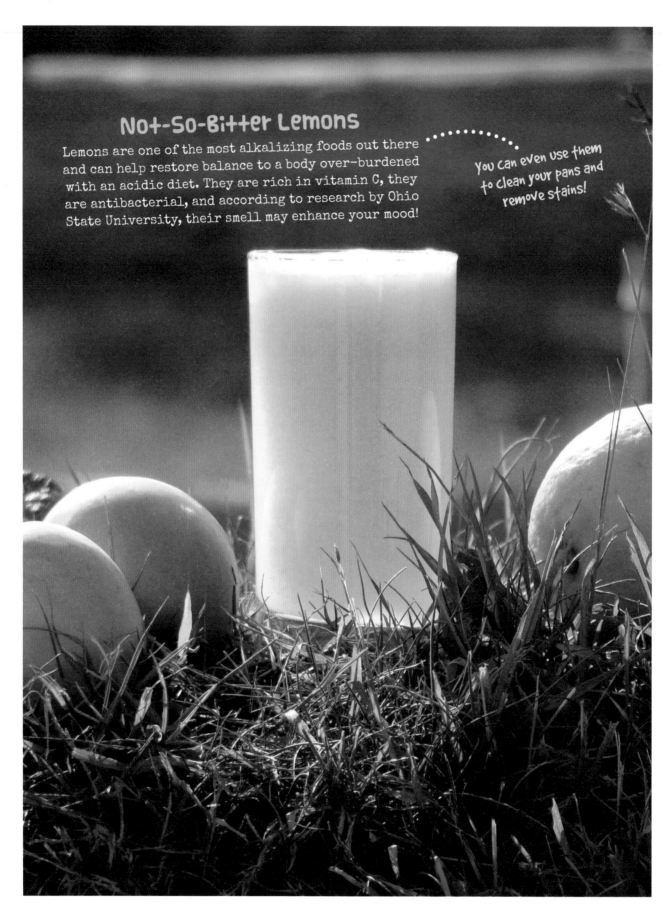

Not-So-Bitter Lemons

Lemons are one of the most alkalizing foods out there and can help restore balance to a body over-burdened with an acidic diet. They are rich in vitamin C, they are antibacterial, and according to research by Ohio State University, their smell may enhance your mood!

You can even use them to clean your pans and remove stains!

Juice Master's World-Famous Lemon . . . Aid

The healthiest, creamiest, scummiest, most natural lemonade in the **whole wide world**!

Golden Delicious Apples
2

Unwaxed Lemon
⅓

Ice Cubes
1 small handful

A Taste Of Childhood Summers

Sandwich the lemon (with the skin on) between the two apples in the chute of the juicer, and juice the lot!

Pour over ice and enjoy!

Best Served... with friends! Why not make a pitcher of this delicious refreshing juice? Using the ratio of two apples and a third of a lemon per person, make a large batch and pour into a jug of crushed ice – perfect for a sizzling summer day!

Time For a Healthy Ice Lolly

Get some empty ice lolly holders, pour in the juice, and pop in the freezer. Makes a gorgeous healthy frosty treat!

Another juicy tip – pour straight into an ice-cube tray and freeze. For a quick and easy smoothie simply add some yogurt, a stack of ice-cubes, blend 'til smooth – you've just created a creamy lemonade!

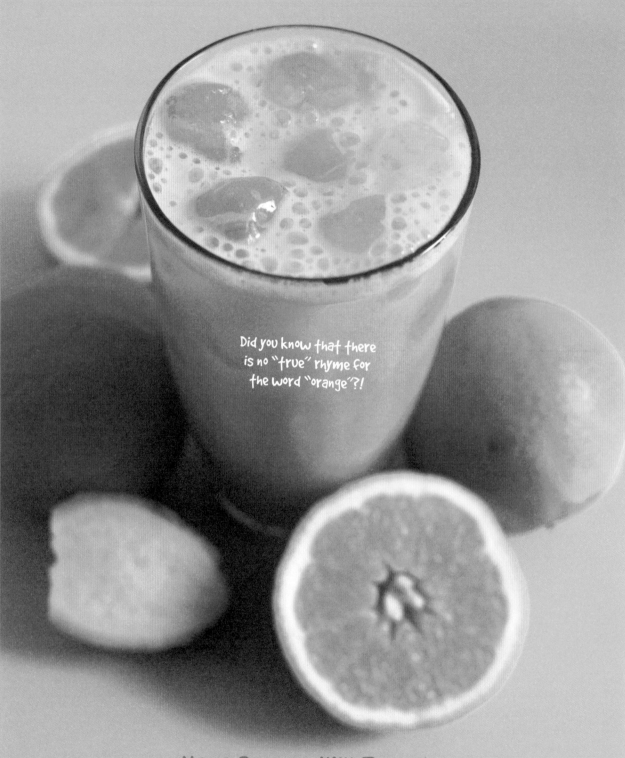

Did you know that there is no "true" rhyme for the word "orange"?!

Have Orange, Will Travel...

Christopher Columbus brought the first orange seeds and seedlings to the New World on his second voyage in 1493. Now the Americas are the largest producer of oranges in the world!

O.J. - with a Kick!

A **spicy twist** on this traditional breakfast juice.

The freshly extracted juice of nature's finest oranges, jazzed up with the slightest hint of real ginger.

Oranges
3 medium (peeled)

Fresh Ginger Root
½ cm chunk

Ice Cubes
1 small handful

Get A Kick Out Of O.J.

Peel the oranges, leaving the as much white pith as possible to make the juice more nutritious and creamier.

Juice all three oranges along with the ginger.

Add some ice to a nice tall glass, slowly pour the juice over, and drink it all up!

Best Served... at breakfast on the terrace at the Marha Beach Club in Turkey, voted in the top 10 places to have breakfast in the world. I have been there, and yes – it is!

A Health Kick!

Of course oranges in this juice are loaded with vitamin C, but the ginger adds an antiviral, antibacterial, antifungal kick!

Fruit With Excellent Taste

It is thought that oranges were cultivated in China as long ago as 2500 B.C. It may have been a hybrid of ancient cultivated origin, possibly between the pomelo and mandarin.

After chocolate and vanilla, orange is the world's favourite flavour!

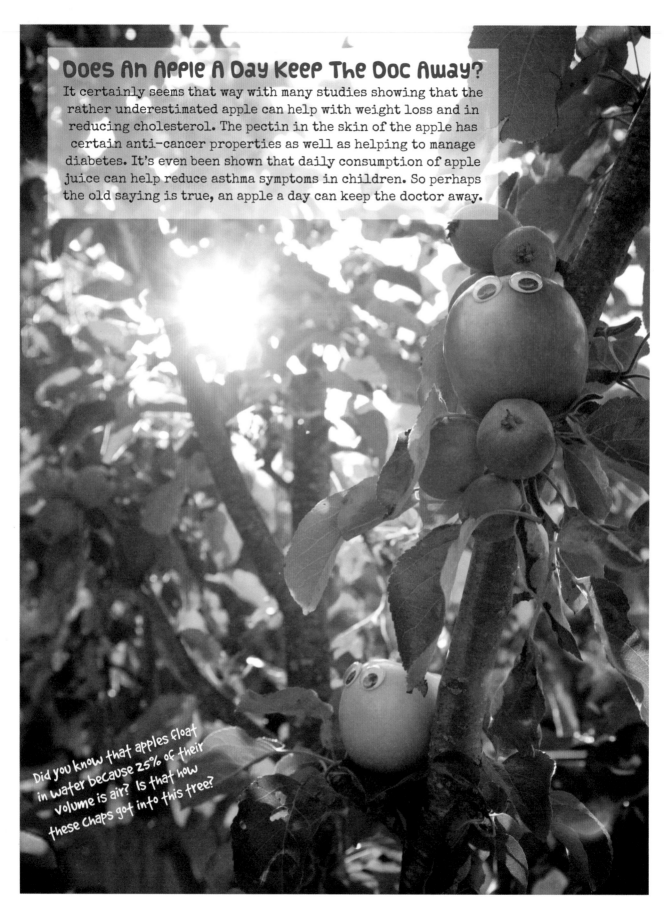

Does An Apple A Day Keep The Doc Away?

It certainly seems that way with many studies showing that the rather underestimated apple can help with weight loss and in reducing cholesterol. The pectin in the skin of the apple has certain anti-cancer properties as well as helping to manage diabetes. It's even been shown that daily consumption of apple juice can help reduce asthma symptoms in children. So perhaps the old saying is true, an apple a day can keep the doctor away.

Did you know that apples float in water because 25% of their volume is air? Is that how these chaps got into this tree?

Golden Delicious

Creamy, delicious pineapple juice and sweet, ripe banana all blended together with a generous chunk of ginger and a splash of lemon. It combines to create **something very special**, that some would call "golden" and (I'm confident) all would say is "delicious".

Pineapple
⅓ medium

Lemon
¼ (peeled)

Golden Delicious Apples
2

Fresh Ginger Root
1 cm chunk

Banana
½ medium (ripe & peeled)

Ice Cubes
1 small handful

Delicious Instructions

Peel the lemon, so the juice is not so sharp, being careful to leave as much of the white pith as you can.

Juice the pineapple (no need to peel if you have a good juicer) with the lemon, apples and ginger. Make sure you sandwich the lemon and ginger between the apples to extract the most juice.

Pour the juice into the blender and add the peeled banana and ice. Blend until smooth and creamy.

Best Served... lying on a deep shag pile rug in front of an open window, with the sunshine flooding in, listening to the mellow sounds of a chilled Ibiza album. Simply allow yourself to drift off into the land of deliciousness…

Apples International

Around the world there are more than 7500 varieties of apple grown. The USA has a whopping 2500 varieties, Red Delicious being the most popular, closely followed by our favourite, the Golden Delicious. Surprising when the only apple that's actually native to the US is the crab-apple (definitely not a good apple to juice). In our humble opinion it's Golden Delicious or Royal Gala.

Some of our Juicy community have even been known to use other apples, including the rather tart Granny Smith!

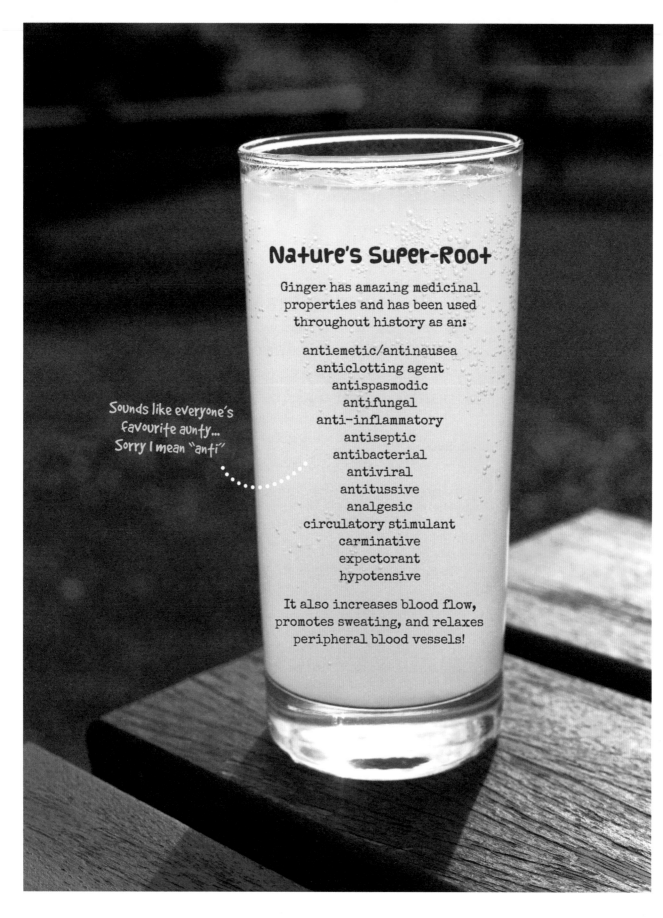

Juice Master's Natural Ginger Beer

Ginger beer is scrummy, but shop bought ginger beer usually has tons of sugar, alcohol, or a combination of the two!

Here's a simple way to make a healthy version at home that is **better than anything** you can get in a shop.

Pellegrino Water
1 litre bottle

Golden Delicious Apple
1

Fresh Ginger Root
1 large claw

Ice Cubes
1 handful

A Refreshing Beverage With Bite

Juice the apple and ginger.

Pour out a small amount of water from a full bottle of Pellegrino – you need to make enough room for the ginger and apple juice.

Pour the juice into the bottle until it's full. Pop the lid on then (gently) shake the bottle to mix.

Once it's settled, pour over ice and enjoy!

Super Secret Identity

Ginger Root isn't even strictly a root – it's a "rhizome", also known as a "creeping rootstock", which is a horizontal stem found underground that sends out roots and shoots from its nodes.

⋮

Too much information? Yeah, I think so too!

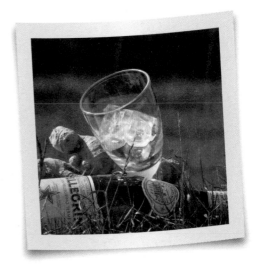

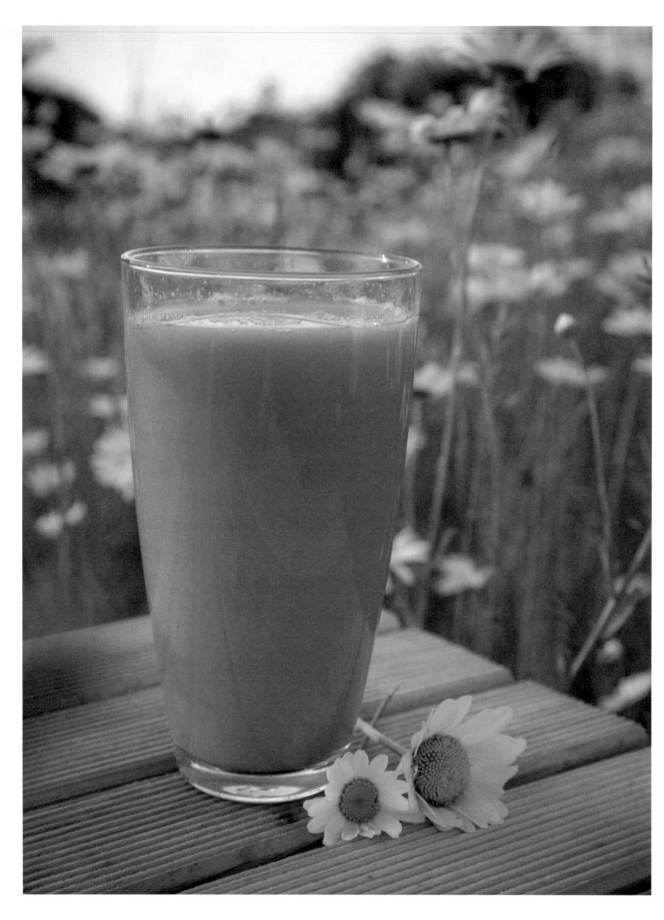

Lip Smackin Mellow Yellow

This lip-smacking smoothie fuses the rich, creaminess of freshly extracted pineapple juice with the zest of lemon, the sweetness of yellow pepper and the calming tones of banana and golden kiwifruit. All blended with ice – taking you *from 60 to mellow* in a few short sips.

Pineapple
½ medium

Gold or Regular Kiwifruit
2 medium (peeled)

Unwaxed Lemon
⅓

Yellow Bell Pepper
½

Golden Delicious Apple
1

Banana
½ (ripe & peeled)

Ice Cubes
1 small handful

Get Those Lips Ready

Peel both of the kiwifruit.

Juice the pineapple (no need to peel if you have a good juicer) with one of the kiwifruit, the lemon (with the skin on), bell pepper and apple.

Put the peeled banana and the other kiwifruit into the blender, along with the ice. Blend until smooth.

Best Served… while listening to yellow submarine. Actually, scrap that! Of all the Beatles songs, Yellow Submarine has to be the worst. What were they on? Maybe the lyrics of Lucy In The Sky With Diamonds is a clue!

No, this is best served whilst wearing your favourite yellow outfit, sitting mellowed-out in a field of beautiful wild daisies. If the sun isn't shining it soon will be!

Kiwifruit Studies

A study at the University of Oslow, Norway found that eating 2–3 kiwifruit per day was as effective as taking aspirin at thinning the blood and preventing clots.

Human studies in Europe and New Zealand found that eating a couple of kiwifruit a day improves the repair of damaged DNA caused by oxidization in the body.

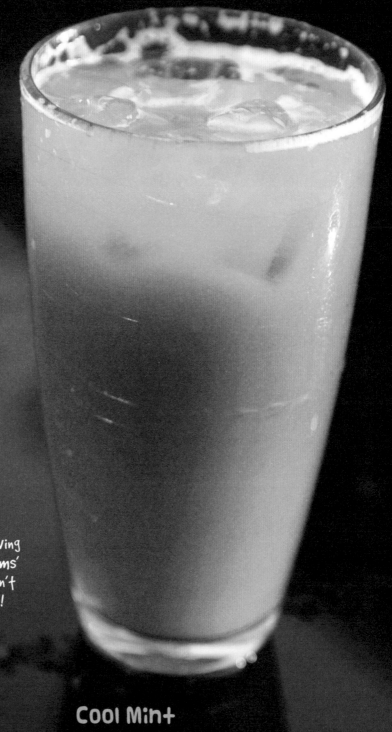

At Juicy HQ we tried shoving mint directly up the teams' noses, but we really didn't see any improvement!

Cool Mint

Recent research conducted at the University of Cincinnati has shown that sniffing mint improves concentration. Several Japanese companies now pipe small amounts through their air-conditioning systems to invigorate workers and improve productivity.

Pineapple, Cucumber & Mint Cooler

Freshly extracted, sweet and creamy pineapple juice, fused with mineral rich cucumber and blended with cool fresh mint and ice.

Pineapple
½ medium

Cucumber
¼ medium

Fresh Mint
1 large handful

Ice Cubes
1 handful

Everybody Be Cool!

Juice the pineapple (no need to peel if you have a good juicer) and cucumber.

Place the mint into the blender, along with the ice. Add the fresh juice and blend for about 60 seconds.

Pour into a nice tall glass, admire and then consume!

Best Served... while lying on a lounger at the Four Seasons in Maui during Whale season – February time(ish). You will see them jumping out of the water as you sip this gorgeous cooling drink. Or you may well have to settle for your kitchen table, but either way, you'll love the juice!

Pineapple Mad

Pineapples are one of the mostly widely exported tropical fruits. Almost a third of the world's production of pineapples and more than half of all canned pineapple comes from Lanai, Hawaii. In fact it's nicknamed "The Pineapple Isle"!

Did you know that, on average, it takes 18 months from planting to harvesting to produce a ripe pineapple fruit?

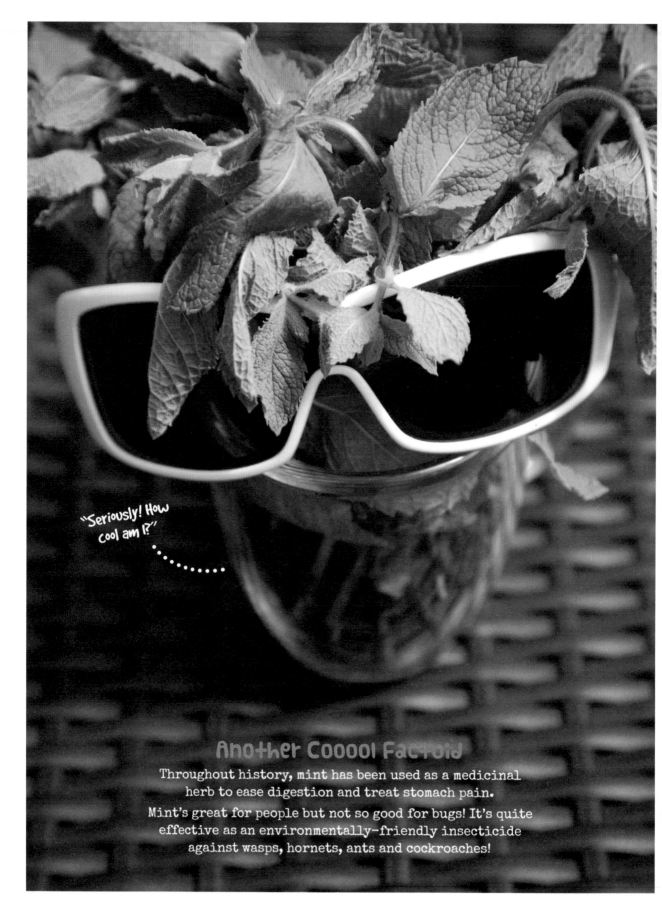

"Seriously! How cool am I?"

Another Coooool Factoid

Throughout history, mint has been used as a medicinal herb to ease digestion and treat stomach pain.

Mint's great for people but not so good for bugs! It's quite effective as an environmentally-friendly insecticide against wasps, hornets, ants and cockroaches!

Apple, Celery & Cool Mint

The *refreshing crisp, cooling tones* of fresh mint, combined with the natural sweetness of delicious apples and cool celery.

Golden Delicious Apples
2

Celery
2 stalks

Fresh Mint
leaves of 4 sprigs

Ice Cubes
1 small handful

Making This Super-cool Juice

Juice the apples and celery.

Next, pour the fresh juice into the blender with the mint leaves and ice, and blend until smooth.

Happy days!

Best Served... as a beautiful cool juice for a hot and sunny day. Picture a tall frosty glass, a big straw, the sun warming your face, you're feeling a bit dozy from the heat and then the refreshing aroma of mint hits you! The cool mintastic taste of the juice wakes up your senses and shakes up your mind. You're ready to take on the world again.

The Big Apple

The largest apple ever picked was grown in Japan and weighed a whopping 1.8 kg (4 lbs 1 oz)!

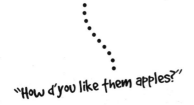

"How d'you like them apples?"

The Weight-Loss Wonder

Just one stalk of celery contains around 10 calories. Some say that it contains "negative calories," which means that it take more calories to digest it than are consumed when you eat it, which is why it's often used as an aid to weight loss.

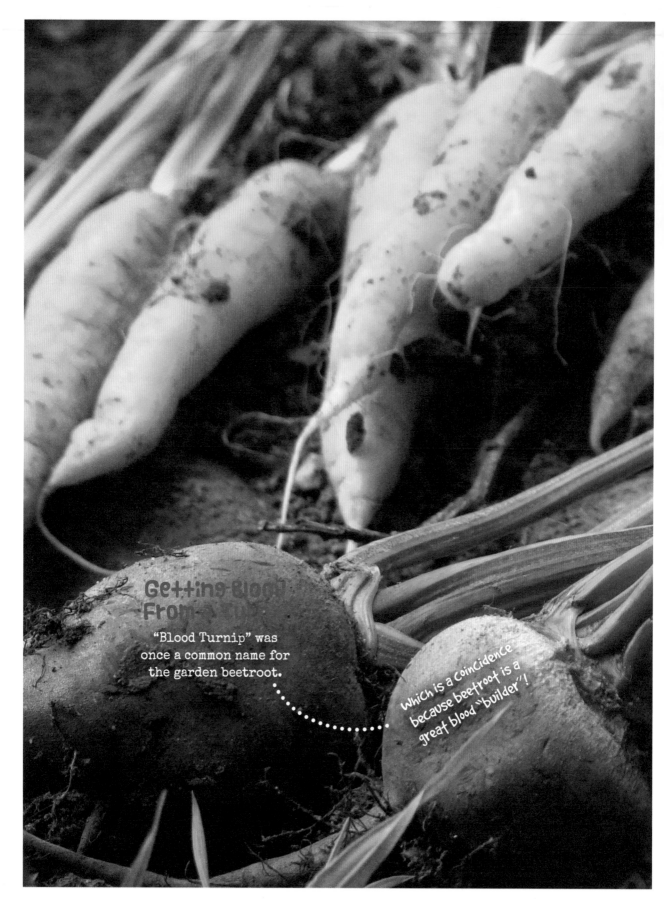

Getting Blood From a Turnip

"Blood Turnip" was once a common name for the garden beetroot.

Which is a coincidence because beetroot is a great blood "builder"!

Apple, Beet, Carrot & Celery

You can't beat a good beet juice! This juice is a little **nutrient powerhouse** and tastes great too! What more could you possibly want?

Golden Delicious Apples
2

Raw Beetroot
1 large

Carrot
1 large

Celery
2 stalks

Ice Cubes
1 handful

How To Make This Ruby Juice

Simply juice the apples, beetroot, carrot and celery, and pour over ice. Easy–peasy!

Best Served... in a large wine glass – and drink this beauty slowly, like a fine wine.

Beet-u-tiful

I'm sure you've already discovered that beetroots have "a lot" of juicy red juice. Not only is this juice a great blood builder, making you glow from the inside. It's also been used to dye fabrics, clothing and even hair a beautiful red colour... and your hands, wooden chopping board and your favourite white shirt!

You have been warned!

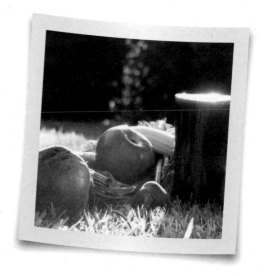

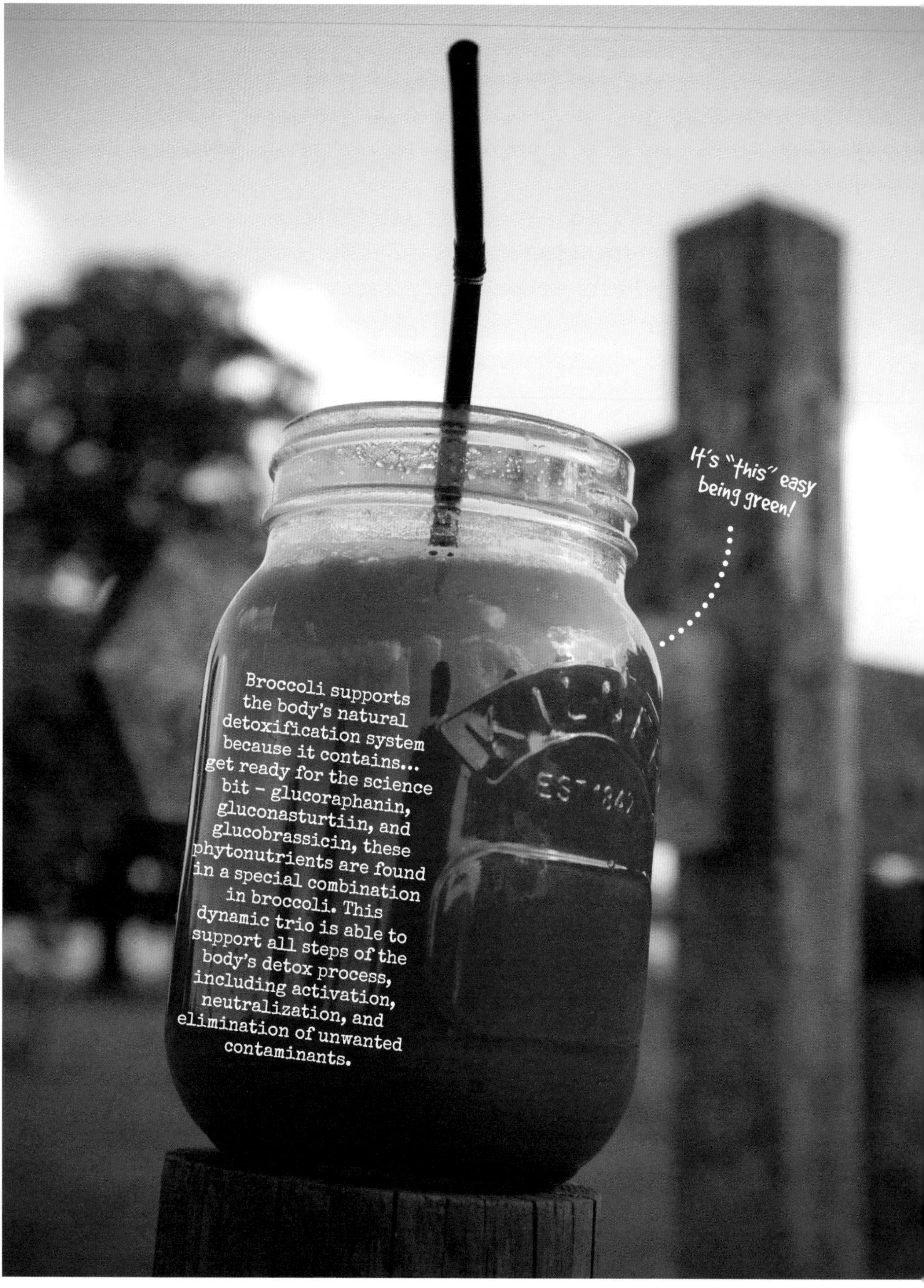

It's "this" easy
being green!

Broccoli supports
the body's natural
detoxification system
because it contains...
get ready for the science
bit – glucoraphanin,
gluconasturtiin, and
glucobrassicin, these
phytonutrients are found
in a special combination
in broccoli. This
dynamic trio is able to
support all steps of the
body's detox process,
including activation,
neutralization, and
elimination of unwanted
contaminants.

Green Superfood

"Superfood" is a term used to describe foods that have a particular high concentration of vitamins or minerals. It could be argued that all fruits and vegetables are indeed "super" foods. After all the humble lemon saved thousands of lives because it cured scurvy – which is **pretty super if you ask me**! However, scientists appear to have separated some fruit and veg from the rest and given them the title of "superfoods".

Golden Delicious Apples
2

Broccoli Stem
3 cm chunk

Celery
½ stalk

Cucumber
¼ medium

Spinach
1 large handful

Unwaxed Lemon
¼

Fresh Ginger Root
1 cm chunk

Ice Cubes
1 small handful

How To Make "Super" In A Glass

Place one apple into the chute of your juicer; behind it tightly pack in the spinach, followed by the lemon, ginger, broccoli, cucumber, celery and the other apple.

Juice the lot and then either pour into a glass over ice or blend with ice in a blender.

Best Served... when you are feeling a little bit like Bridget Jones on a bad day but instead of reaching for the ice cream and cookies, you decide to inject some super food into your system and make yourself feel super healthy instead of super sick! Just a thought...

See Why Broccoli Is So Super

Broccoli is a gold mine (or should we say "green"mine) of nutrition. This green gem can be good for your sight. The carotenoid lutein in broccoli can help prevent age-related macular degeneration and cataracts. Broccoli is also a good source of vitamin A which is needed to form retinal, the light-absorbing molecule that is essential for both low-light and colour vision.

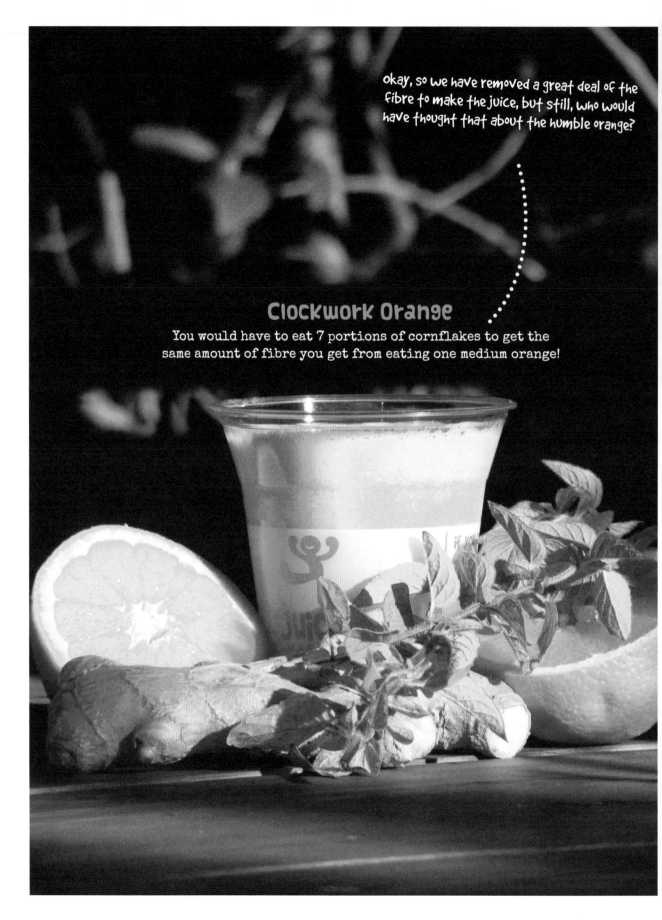

okay, so we have removed a great deal of the fibre to make the juice, but still, who would have thought that about the humble orange?

Clockwork Orange

You would have to eat 7 portions of cornflakes to get the same amount of fibre you get from eating one medium orange!

Orange, Mint & Ginger Zinger

Gorgeous freshly extracted, creamy orange juice, with a hint of fresh ginger, blended with cooling mint and ice.

Oranges
4 medium (peeled)

Fresh Ginger Root
1 cm chunk

Fresh Mint
1 large handful

Ice Cubes
1 small handful

Time For A Zing

Peel the oranges leaving as much of the white pith as possible for a creamier and more nutrient rich juice.

Juice the oranges and the ginger.

Place the mint into your blender, along with ice add the fresh juice. Blend for about 60 seconds, pour and enjoy!

Best Served... lying in the park with friends on a beautiful day, after a good old game of rounders (if you are in America you call it "baseball" and take it far too seriously!). If that's not possible, simply serve in a gorgeous glass.

Oranges With Appeal

Hesperetin and naringenin are flavonoids found in citrus fruits. Naringenin is found to have a bio-active effect on human health as an antioxidant, free radical scavenger, anti-inflammatory, and immune system modulator. It also been shown to reduce oxidant injury to DNA in vitro studies.

Oranges With No A-peel

The oils in orange skin are indigestible, but the pith is where most of the nutrients are found. So when juicing oranges remember: no skin, just pith makes the juice creamier and healthier!

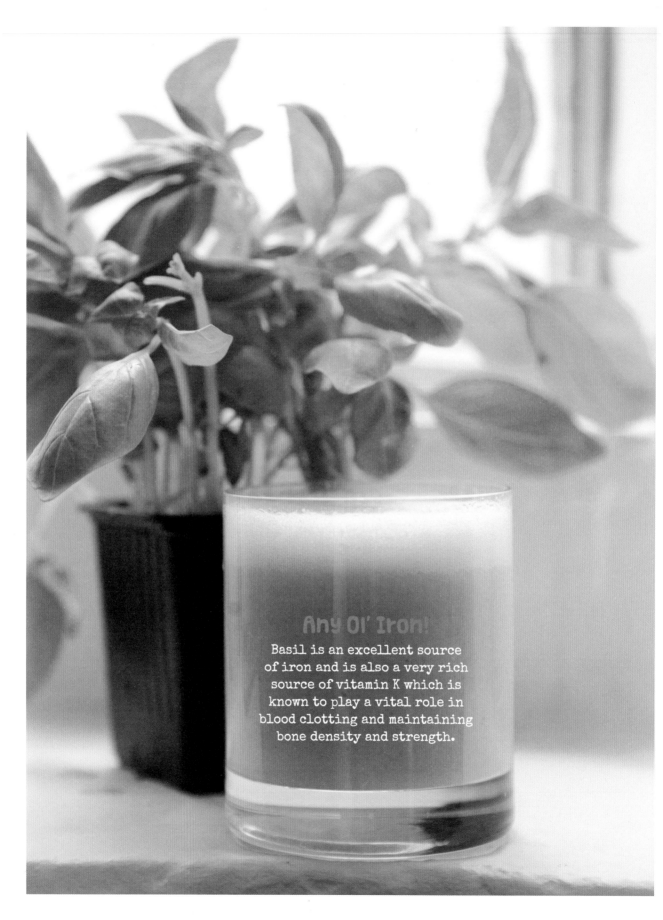

Any Ol' Iron!

Basil is an excellent source
of iron and is also a very rich
source of vitamin K which is
known to play a vital role in
blood clotting and maintaining
bone density and strength.

Basil Lush!

You won't often see Basil making its way into a Juice
Master smoothie, but there is a first time for everything,
and once you've tasted it, you'll be glad it did!

Pineapple
1 small

Lime
1 (peeled)

Mango
1 small (ripe, peeled & pitted)

Fresh Basil
leaves from 4 sprigs

Bio Live Yogurt
3 tablespoons

Ice Cubes
1 small handful

Boom! Boom!

Peel the lime, leaving as much of the white pith as possible – it's where most of the nutrients are.

Juice the pineapple (no need to peel if you have a good juicer) and lime.

Carefully slice the mango just off-centre down both sides, avoiding the large stone inside, then scoop out the flesh from the skin and add to the blender.

Add the basil, yogurt (if you are a vegan, just leave this out or use soya yogurt) and ice, then blend until smooth.

Best Served... anytime – anywhere!

See what I've done there? With the "Basil" and "Brush" thing? oh, never mind...

Brush Up on Some Basil Facts

Scientific studies have established that compounds in basil oil have potent antioxidant, antiviral and antimicrobial properties and have potential in cancer treatments.

Basil also is quite a good mosquito repellant!

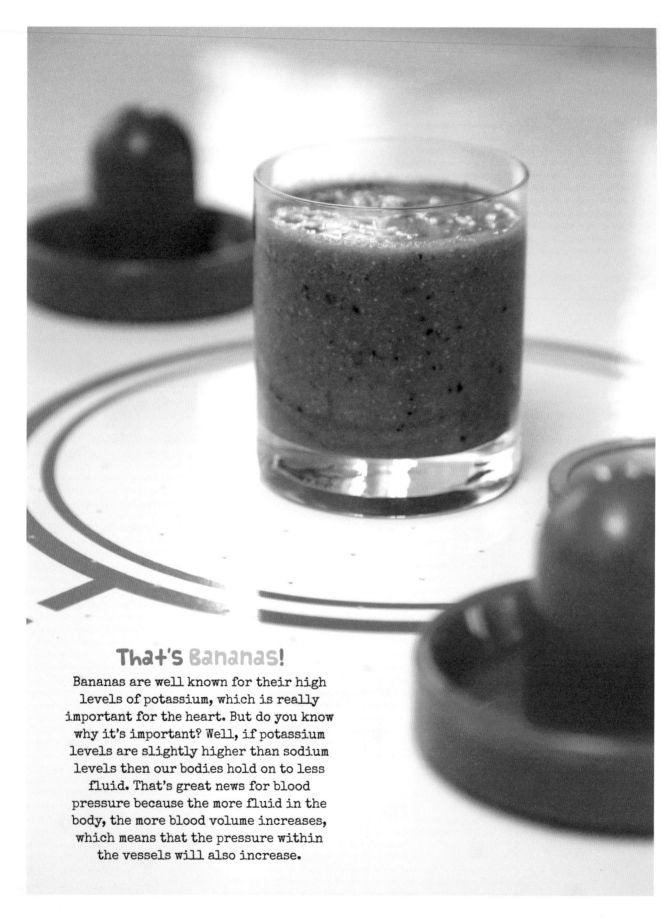

That's Bananas!

Bananas are well known for their high
levels of potassium, which is really
important for the heart. But do you know
why it's important? Well, if potassium
levels are slightly higher than sodium
levels then our bodies hold on to less
fluid. That's great news for blood
pressure because the more fluid in the
body, the more blood volume increases,
which means that the pressure within
the vessels will also increase.

Fruit 'n' Nut

Fruit and nuts is just one of those terrific combinations that works in **perfect taste synergy**. The sweet flavours of the fruity berries are balanced by the dense, rich nuts. In contrast the heaviness of the nuts is lifted by the juiciness of the berries. This is nature working in true harmony. However, unlike the popular chocolate bar that hijacked Mother Nature's amazing invention, this smoothie is 100% pure, 100% natural and 100% guilt free!

Raw Brazil Nuts
3 (unsalted)

Raw Almonds
3 (unsalted)

Banana
½ medium (ripe)

Golden Delicious Apples
3

Seasonal Mixed Berries
1 large handful (fresh or frozen)

Raisins
1 small handful

Ice Cubes
1 small handful

Everyone's A Fruit & Nut-Case

Make sure you choose "raw" nuts not the roasted ones and leave the salt off, it won't go well with the juice!

Juice the apples and pour into the blender.

Add the nuts, raisins, peeled banana and berries to the blender and blend until very smooth (you don't want to be *eating* the nuts!)

Best Served... when you would normally be reaching for a Cadbury's Fruit & Nut bar. This gorgeous smoothie is sweet and extremely filling, but not an artificial ingredient in sight. If you really feel the need for a choc fix, you can always add some good quality high cocoa content fair-trade chocolate to the blender... but only if you really have to!

That's Nuts!

Brazil nuts are exceptionally high in the trace mineral selenium, which is fantastic for the immune system and for managing inflammation in the body.

Ahoy Me Limey! Limes are a great source of vitamin C and were used by British sailors as a way of preventing scurvy in the 1800s. They're not just good to eat — their essence is used in perfumes, cleaning products and aromatherapy. And in Tantra it is even believed they can repel evil spirits!

The Green Goddess

Deliciously thick conference pear juice, complemented with the sharp juice from a ripe lime, calmed with nutrient rich spinach and celery juice, cooled with fresh cucumber and sweetened with pure apple juice.

Golden Delicious Apple
1

Spinach
1 small handful

Conference Pear
1

Unwaxed Lime
1

Celery
1 stalk

Cucumber
¼ medium

Ice Cubes
1 small handful

Put Them All Together Like This

Place the apple into the chute of the juicer and then pack the spinach in tightly behind it. Add the pear, lime and celery, cucumber and juice the lot.

Best Served...
on an empty stomach, in a wine glass over ice and consumed 30 minutes before you do that Ashtanga Yoga session you promised yourself – or not perhaps!

Did You Know?

There are two main varieties of lime – Key and Persian.

Limes are not only good for you but their extracts are used in cleaning products!

"As cool as a cucumber" was first used in a poem by John Gay, entitled "New Song on New Similes" in 1732 (just after half past five!) in the line: "I... cool as a cucumber could see the rest of Womankind."

Yes, we at Juicy HQ were rather hoping the origin of this phrase was slightly more exciting!

Where better to enjoy this than overlooking the mountains at the Juice Master Rustic Retreat?!

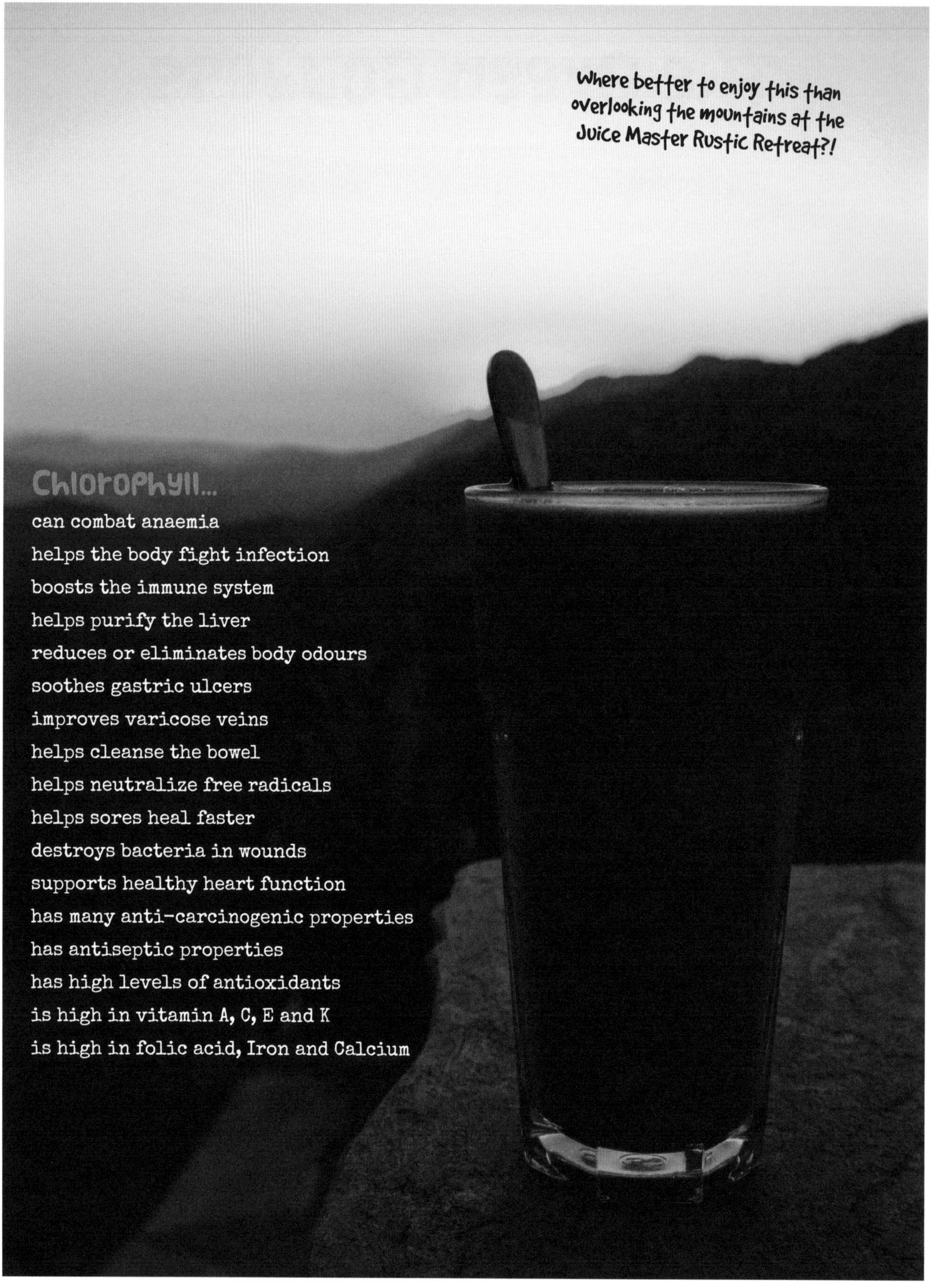

Chlorophyll...

can combat anaemia
helps the body fight infection
boosts the immune system
helps purify the liver
reduces or eliminates body odours
soothes gastric ulcers
improves varicose veins
helps cleanse the bowel
helps neutralize free radicals
helps sores heal faster
destroys bacteria in wounds
supports healthy heart function
has many anti-carcinogenic properties
has antiseptic properties
has high levels of antioxidants
is high in vitamin A, C, E and K
is high in folic acid, Iron and Calcium

Chlorophyll Power

Going "green" is all the rage and people are doing their bit to stop polluting the planet. And if you "pollute" your inner environment too, you will cause damage – sometimes irreversibly.

Chlorophyll is the pigment found in all green plants that allows the plant to capture the sun's energy (photosynthesis). Chlorophyll is nearly identical to the oxygen-carrying haemoglobin in your blood and is totally amazing when it comes to **optimum health**.

With that in mind, it's really worth getting some of this green juice inside you every day!

Pineapple
½ medium

Cucumber
¼ medium

Lime
½ (peeled)

Celery
½ stalk

Spinach
1 handful

Green Leafy Vegetables
1 handful (kale + cabbage + watercress)

Broccoli Stem
3 cm chunk

Ice Cubes
1 small handful

How To Create

Peel the lime, leaving as much of the white pith as possible – it's where most of the nutrients are.

Juice the pineapple (no need to peel if you have a good juicer) and all the other ingredients. Make sure you pack the spinach and leafy vegetables tightly into the chute of the juicer, before juicing, to extract the most juice.

Pour over ice and get ready to feel the power!

For an extra dose of chlorophyll add a small teaspoon of wheatgrass powder or spirulina – it takes it up several levels! If you can do a wheatgrass shot – even better! If you're adding spirulina or wheatgrass powder then you will need to whizz it all up in the blender before drinking.

Best Served... at the Juice Master Rustic Retreat – of course! It's a place of health, relaxation and beautiful views. Or perhaps you could have this green powerhouse on the go.

A Fact To Remember

Numerous studies have found that some purple fruits and veg may be good for your memory. Blueberries contain anthocyanin – a known "memory boosting" phytochemical – as well as many other phytochemicals that contribute to healthy brain function. Beetroots are also a good source of anthocyanin and folic acid. So if your brain is feeling a little weary this boost of purple fruit and veg should be very beneficial.

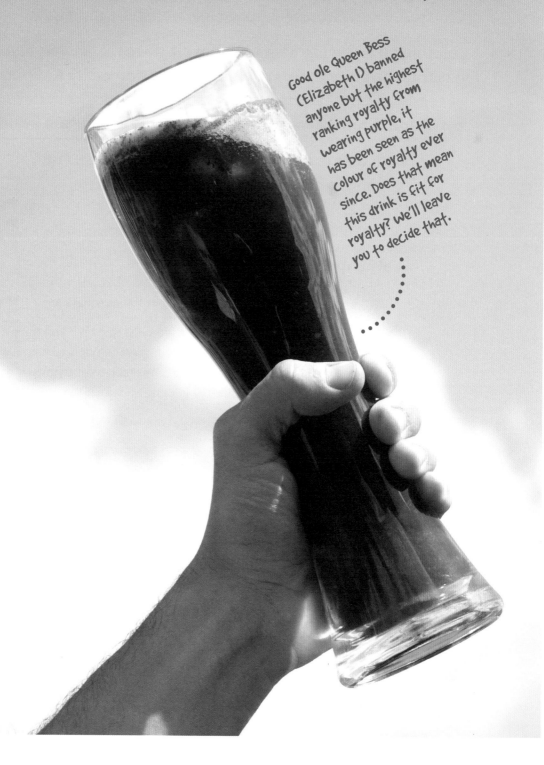

Good ole Queen Bess (Elizabeth I) banned anyone but the highest ranking royalty from wearing purple, it has been seen as the colour of royalty ever since. Does that mean this drink is fit for royalty? We'll leave you to decide that.

Pure Purple Power

Delicious, dark, deep blueberries and blackberries combined with the sweet crimson tones of fresh beetroot juice and pure, freshly extracted apple juice.

Rich in antioxidants and with vitamins A, B, C, and K, plus calcium, magnesium, iron and phosphorous – this smoothie is **not just a pretty colour**. It's also nice to get the goodness of blueberries without a muffin in sight!

Golden Delicious Apples
2

Raw Beetroot
1

Blueberries
1 handful

Blackberries
1 handful

Ice Cubes
1 small handful

How To Create

Juice the apples and beetroot.

Pour the fresh juice into the blender. Add the blueberries, blackberries and ice and blend.

Best Served... chilling out on a large sofa, listening to the breathtaking voice of Beverly Knight singing her version of George Michael's One More Try...

The Colour Purple

Blueberries are true kings of the fruit world and have quite a majestic reputation due to their many health properties. They are so renowned for their very high antioxidant capacity. The blue/purple pigment is created by a special group of chemicals called anthocyanidins. These help to protect tissue against oxidative damage in the body which is associated with almost every disease at some level or another.

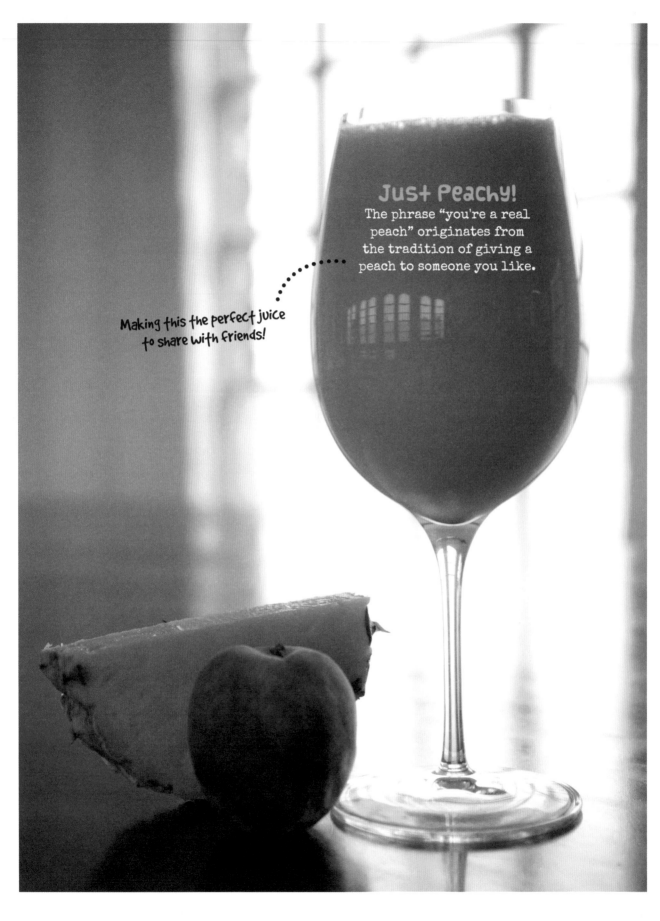

Just Peachy!
The phrase "you're a real peach" originates from the tradition of giving a peach to someone you like.

Making this the perfect juice to share with friends!

Peaches & Cream

Perfectly delicious peaches make this divinely creamy, smooth and absolutely yummy smoothie. Blended with the sweetness of pineapple juice and softened with a touch of bio-live yogurt, this is a **sensation on the taste buds**!

Pineapple
1 medium

Peaches
3 (ripe & pitted)

Bio-Live Yogurt
200 ml

Ice Cubes
1 small handful

A Little Taste Of Heaven

Juice the pineapple (no need to peel if you have a good juicer).

Remove the stone from the peaches and place them into the blender. Pour in the fresh juice, yogurt and ice. Blend until creamy.

Best Served... lying on the front of a yacht in the Med in your swim wear, while the sun warms every inch of your body. If that is not possible, close your eyes wherever you are as you take a sip of this ridiculously gorgeous smoothie and allow your imagination to drift...

Know Your Peaches

Peaches are divided into "clingstones" that have flesh that sticks to the stones but are soft, sweet and juicy; "freestones" that are not as sweet but easier to eat from your hands as the flesh doesn't cling to the stones; and "semi-freestones" which have been bred to combine the best of both.

Peach flowers have a mild sedative effect and are good for restless children, especially when boiled in water with a little honey.

Just to be clear you should be boiling the flowers not the children!

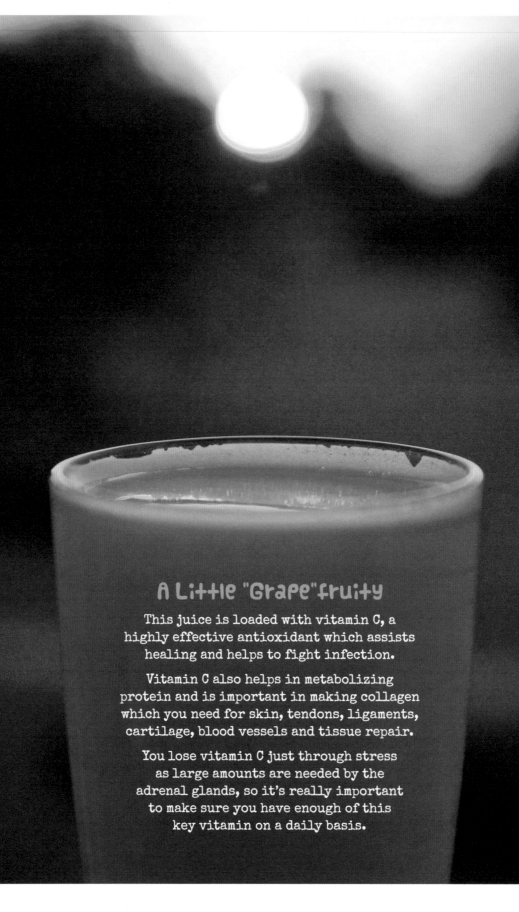

A Little "Grape"fruity

This juice is loaded with vitamin C, a
highly effective antioxidant which assists
healing and helps to fight infection.

Vitamin C also helps in metabolizing
protein and is important in making collagen
which you need for skin, tendons, ligaments,
cartilage, blood vessels and tissue repair.

You lose vitamin C just through stress
as large amounts are needed by the
adrenal glands, so it's really important
to make sure you have enough of this
key vitamin on a daily basis.

Sunset Sparkle

Rich, sweet and deliciously creamy pineapple juice, given a bite with the sharpness of freshly extracted ginger juice, complemented beautifully with the slight bitterness of pink grapefruit, and all jazzed up with the fizz of naturally carbonated mineral water then cooled with ice.

We **love** this at juicy HQ!

Pineapple
⅓ medium

Pink Grapefruit
1 medium (peeled)

Fresh Ginger Root
1 cm chunk

Sparkling Mineral Water
1 small bottle

Ice Cubes
1 small handful

Are you Ready to Sparkle?

Peel the grapefruit, leaving the white pith to make the juice more nutritious.

Juice the pineapple (no need to peel if you have a good juicer) with the grapefruit and ginger.

Pour the fresh juice into a glass over ice until two-thirds full. Top-up with the sparkling water.

Best Served... after a sunset surf in Cornwall, Portugal or Hawaii. That beautiful free feeling that only snow-boarding or surfing can give you – sun just going down, waves just right and floating with your thoughts "out back" with the evening sun beating on your face. This drink is just perfect for when you get out and watch the sun go down in your wet-suit. Make and place in a flask and take to beach…

Mineral Water

Crystal clear, pure and refreshing, mineral water has been associated with healing for centuries. Mineral water is usually taken directly from its source. A world famous source of mineral rich water is the beautiful city of "Bath" in Somerset, amazingly it's been used since Roman times.

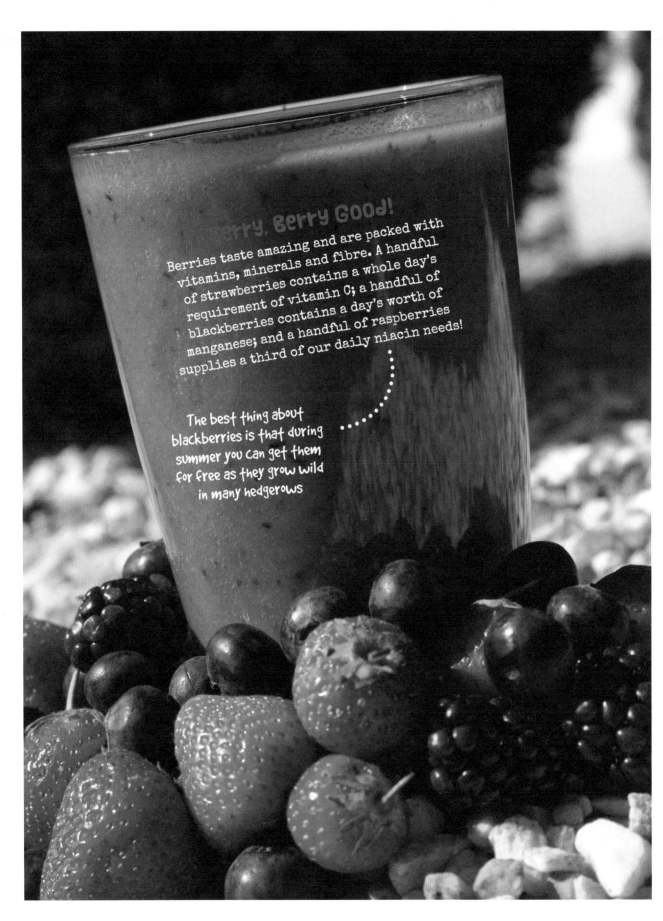

Berry, Berry Good!

Berries taste amazing and are packed with vitamins, minerals and fibre. A handful of strawberries contains a whole day's requirement of vitamin C; a handful of blackberries contains a day's worth of manganese; and a handful of raspberries supplies a third of our daily niacin needs!

The best thing about blackberries is that during summer you can get them for free as they grow wild in many hedgerows

Mixed Seed & Berry Smoothie

Sweet succulent mixed berries blended with creamy apple juice, bio-live yogurt and then naturally fortified with a generous sprinkling of mixed seeds, **loaded with essential fatty acids**.

Golden Delicious Apples
2

Blueberries
1 handful

Blackberries
1 handful

Raspberries
1 handful

Strawberries
1 handful

Bio-Live Yogurt
1 tablespoon

Mixed Seeds
1 tablespoon

Ice Cubes
1 handful

How To Mix It Up

Mixed seeds are often found ready-mixed in a small bag from most supermarkets, usually consisting of sunflower, pumpkin, sesame and others.

Juice the apples and pour into the blender.

Add all the berries, yogurt, seeds and ice and blend for a just a few seconds. Don't forget: if you use frozen berries there is no need to add extra ice to the blender.

Best Served... lying in a hot bubble bath after a hard day at work, Nora Jones on the playlist, candles flickering, sipping your Mixed Seed Berry Smoothie from a chilled wine goblet... novel or magazine in hand... bliss!

Small But Powerful

Seeds may be tiny, but they are almighty in terms of nutrition. They are a fantastic source of protein, dietary fibre, omega-3 fatty acids and phytonutrients.

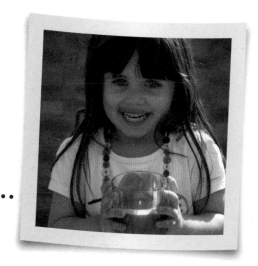

This is little Ruby with ruby lips... Made more ruby by the ruby coloured drink!

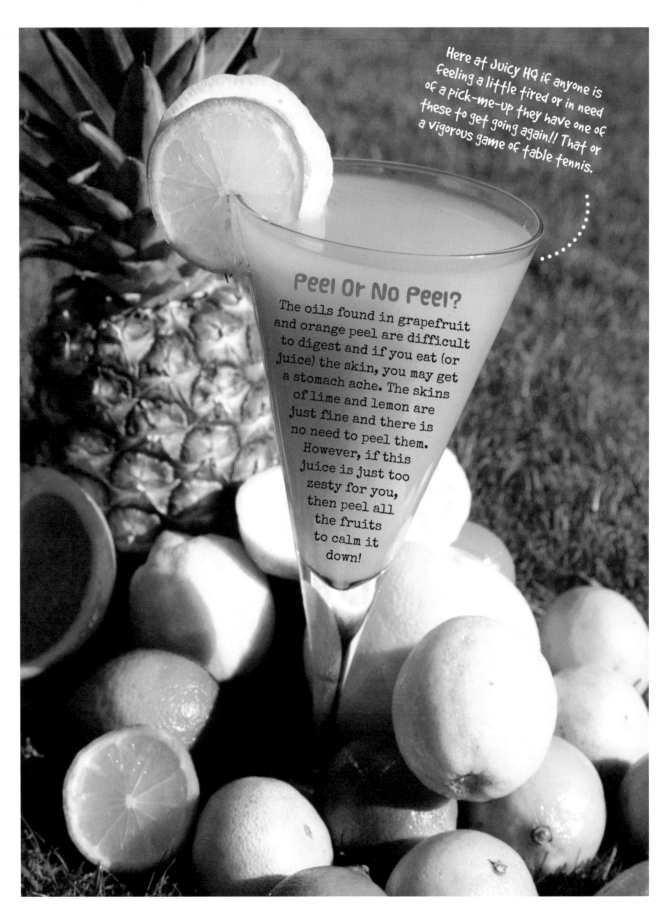

Here at Juicy HQ if anyone is feeling a little tired or in need of a pick-me-up they have one of these to get going again!! That or a vigorous game of table tennis.

Peel Or No Peel?

The oils found in grapefruit and orange peel are difficult to digest and if you eat (or juice) the skin, you may get a stomach ache. The skins of lime and lemon are just fine and there is no need to peel them. However, if this juice is just too zesty for you, then peel all the fruits to calm it down!

Super Sharp & Super Zesty

If you are looking for a juice that will slap you around the face, this is it! If you remember the "You've Been Tango'd" adverts from yesteryear, you'll recall the little orange man who came up to the guy who had just drunk his Tango and slapped him around the face.

This zingy, zesty juice will feel like that... well it won't hurt you like a slap in the face, but it'll **wake you and your senses up** for sure.

Pink Grapefruit
½ medium (peeled)

Orange
1 (peeled)

Pineapple
¼ medium

Unwaxed Lime
½

Unwaxed Lemon
½

Ice Cubes
1 small handful

How To Make This Zesty Juice

Peel the grapefruit and orange, leaving as much of the white pith as possible. There is no need to peel the lime or lemon.

Juice the orange, lemon, lime and grapefruit followed by the pineapple (no need to peel if you have a good juicer).

Pour over ice and enjoy.

Best Served... You know when you realize you need to totally blitz your house and give it a spring clean? Well, make this juice before you start, and then when you're all done reward a morning of hard work by jumping onto your giant sofa with this super zesty juice. It will smell as good as your freshly cleaned house.

Waxing Lyrical

Most lemons and limes these days are "waxed" because big supermarkets want them to look all shiny and appealing on their shelves. If I wanted to eat wax I would chew on a candle. So if you can't get hold of "unwaxed" lemons and limes, make sure you give them a good scrub or peel them first.

Rich in Redness

Blood oranges contain the antioxidant anthocyanin – which is part of the reason they have red flesh. It's been linked with helping to reduce heart disease, several types of cancer and it also helps to maintain a healthy cholesterol count. Studies also suggest that this antioxidant can help reduce the risk of cataracts and to speed up the body's natural healing process. So, not much then!

Warning! Don't get any blood orange juice on that nice white shirt of yours, it may never come out!

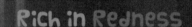

Sunrise Sensation

Start your day the right way with this delicious, creamy pink grapefruit juice combined with Florida's finest "blood" orange juice, blended with some thick natural yogurt and a sweet fair-trade banana.

Breakfast doesn't get tastier than this!

Pink Grapefruit
½ (peeled)

Florida Blood Oranges
2 (peeled)

Banana
1 medium (ripe & peeled)

Bio-live Yogurt
3 heaped tablespoons

Ice Cubes
1 small handful

Good Morning, Sunshine!

Peel the rosy red grapefruit and oranges leaving as much of the white pith as possible for a more nutritious and much creamier tasting juice.

Juice the grapefruit and oranges.

Pour the fresh juice into the blender and add the banana, yogurt and ice. Blend until smooth.

Best Served... in the morning sun, maybe sitting on a white painted porch looking out at the sun rising over some golden fields, listening to the birds singing and breathing in the fresh morning air... ready to start having a great day?

Why Blood oranges?

Apart from looking rather stunning, blood oranges are high in vitamins C and A, calcium, thiamine, and folic acid. The level of vitamins (particularly vitamin C) contained within blood oranges is higher than other oranges.

What About The Grapefruit?

Grapefruits are a great source of vitamin C. One-half of a grapefruit provides all the vitamin C your body needs for the day. Studies have found that grapefruit helps reduce cholesterol and contains spermidine, which has been found to help human immune cells live longer.

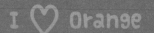

I ♡ Orange

A study from Wageningen University, in the Netherlands, found that orange fruit and veg are best for protecting the heart and preventing fatty build-ups in the arteries.

The diets of 20,000 men and women were examined, noting the amount of green, orange, yellow, red, purple and white fruit and vegetables. Carrots were the largest contributor in the orange group and were associated with a massive 32% lower risk of heart disease.

With a rainbow of natural colours in this juice, you can rest assured your cells will be getting a tremendous balance of nutrition and protection.

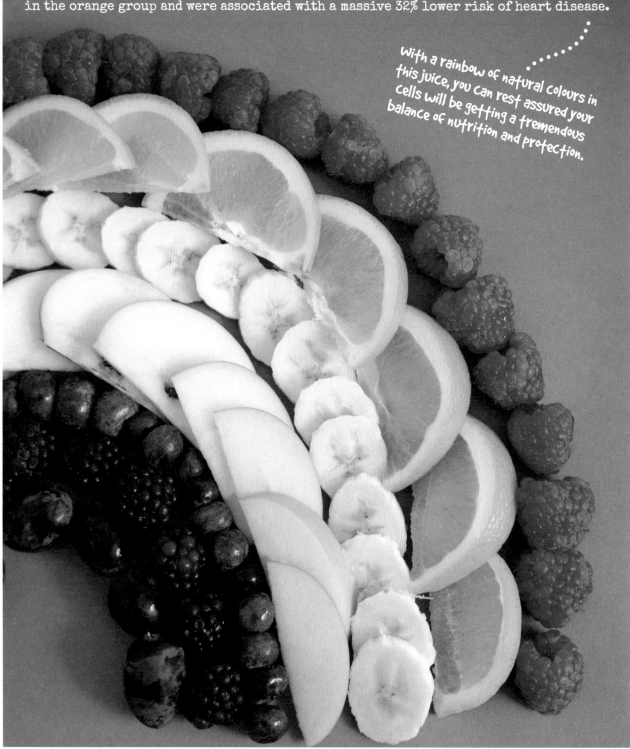

Over The Rainbow

One thing health "experts" appear to agree on is that we need a spectrum of different coloured fruit and veg in our diets. Each distinctive colour holds its very own unique combination of nutritional coding that feeds and heals the body. With the rainbow of natural colours in this juice, you can rest assured your cells will be getting a tremendous *balance of nutrition and protection*.

Red **Raspberries**
1 small handful

Orange
1 (peeled)

Yellow **Banana**
½ medium (ripe & peeled)

Green **Apples**
2

Blue**berries**
1 small handful

Indigo **Blackberries**
1 small handful

Violet **Seedless Grapes**
1 small bunch

Ice Cubes
1 small handful

Up Above The Streets & Houses

Peel the orange, leaving the white pith – it's where most of the nutrients live!

Juice the apples, orange and grapes. Make sure you pack the orange and grapes tightly into the chute of the juicer, between the apples, to extract the most juice.

Pour the fresh juice into the blender. Add the raspberries, peeled banana, blueberries, blackberries and ice, and then blend.

We appreciate it went in a rainbow of colours and came out a bit brown, but your body will most certainly thank you for this delicious burst of rainbow goodness!

Best Served... watching the wonderful Judy Garland singing "Somewhere Over The Rainbow" in the timeless classic *The Wizard Of Oz*! Or better still while watching a real rainbow over the lake at Juicy Oasis Health Retreat & Spa as you sit on the Juice Terrace with like-minded people chatting away about happy things.

If you can't remember what order the colours of a rainbow go in remember "Raspberries of York Give Body Incredible Vitality."

Breakfast Shake, 'Chillin on the beautiful white sand of St Ives beach... In delicious Cornwall

The Ultimate Fruit Breakfast Shake

They say that breakfast is the most important meal of the day and I feel it's vital to get it right. Mornings are without question the best time to get freshly extracted juice into your system. This shake is wonderful for all the family and you won't need anything else – it should be your *entire* breakfast. It's **tasty, nutritious and extremely filling** without leaving you feeling bloated. You'll be good 'til lunch!

Oranges
3 medium (peeled)

Lime
1 (peeled)

Muesli
3 heaped teaspoons

Bio-Live Yogurt
3 tablespoons

Banana
1 (ripe & peeled)

Berries (Your Choice)
1 small handful

Cinnamon
large pinch

Ice Cubes
1 handful

Make This Fruity Shake

For this recipe you should get a really good quality muesli – one that is loaded with fruit, nuts, seeds, oats and no added sugar, artificial sweeteners, flavours or colours. There are many great mueslis these days and as you are only using a couple of tablespoons full, it's worth getting the very best!

Peel and juice the oranges and the lime, remembering to leave as much white pith as you can.

Place the muesli, yogurt, banana, berries, ice and pinch of cinnamon into the blender. Blend until smooth. Because of the nuts in the muesli you may need to blend for more than a minute depending on your blender. If you really like cinnamon you can add a small pinch on top after you have poured into a gorgeous glass (like they do with a cappuccino).

Best Served... sitting on the bar stools around the breakfast bar with an early episode of Friends on the TV or listening to the one and only Chris Evans on BBC Radio 2 or if you are a little more frantic, Chris Moyles on Radio 1. And you never know, by the time you read this he may have even come up with some new content and have ditched "Car Park Catchphrase" and the "Tedious Link"... but as he's used it for over 10 years I doubt it!

Fun Mango Facts

Mango is a rich source of potassium which helps to control heart rate and blood pressure, as well as being a good source of vitamins A, B6, C, E and K, iron, copper, magnesium and manganese – try saying all that in one breath!

And believe it or not, they're actually distantly related to pistachios and cashews!

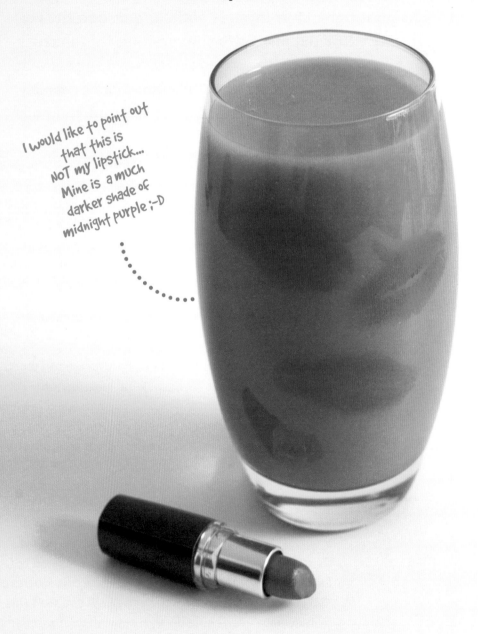

I would like to point out that this is NOT my lipstick... Mine is a much darker shade of midnight purple ;-D

Sun "Kissed" Shake

All of the ingredients in this creamy, sweet smoothie have been **"kissed" by the sun**. Mouth-wateringly delicious, freshly extracted mango juice, combined with orange and pineapple juice and a squeeze of lime. All blended with freshly picked strawberries. Nice one "sun"!

Pineapple
¼ large

Mango
½ large (ripe, peeled & pitted)

Orange
1 medium (peeled)

Lime
½

Strawberries
1 handful

Ice Cubes
1 small handful

Pucker up!

Peel the orange, keeping as much of the white pith as possible. Carefully slice the mango just off-centre, avoiding the large stone inside, then scoop out the flesh from the skin.

Juice the pineapple (no need to peel if you have a good juicer), mango and orange.

Pour the fresh juice into the blender with the strawberries, ice and squeeze in the lime. Blend until smooth.

Best Served... on a large blanket, on a grass embankment, overlooking the Thames (perhaps Richmond), watching the sun reflected on the water as you feel its warmth on your body. Now of course the chances of there being any sun in the UK is extremely rare, so make sure you time it right – I believe summer is on June 21st and lasts for approximately one day – enjoy!

Mangoes Into A Bar & Discovers .... These Facts!

Mango is nutritionally very rich! It's an excellent source of vitamin A and flavonoids including beta-carotene, alpha-carotene, and beta-cryptoxanthin, when together they are known to have antioxidant properties and are also essential for vision. Vitamin A is also needed for maintaining healthy mucus membranes and skin.

Mango is also a great source of Vitamin B6 (pyridoxine) which controls homocysteine levels in the blood, which may otherwise be harmful to blood vessels and cause heart disease and strokes.

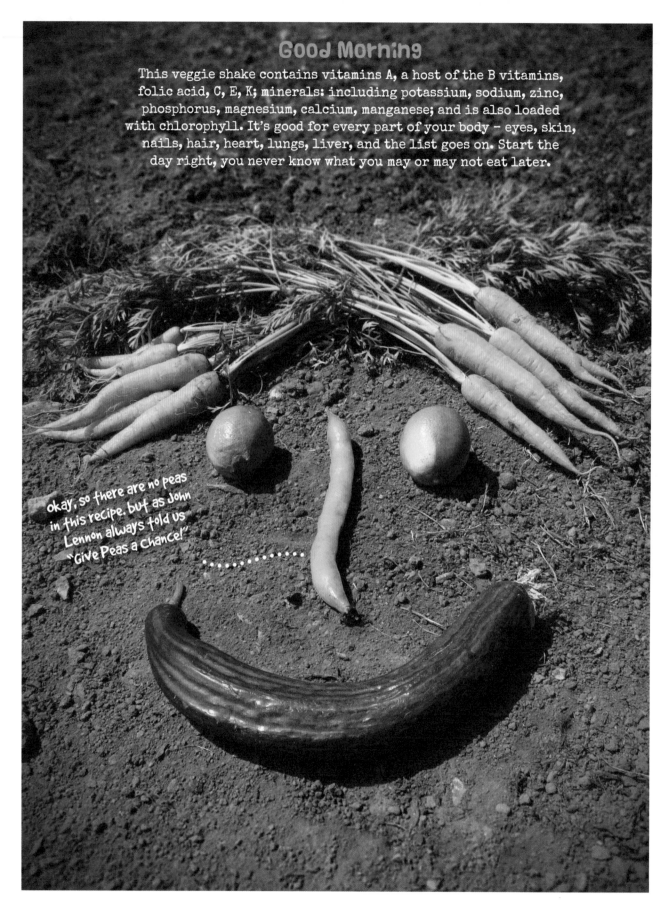

Good Morning

This veggie shake contains vitamins A, a host of the B vitamins, folic acid, C, E, K; minerals: including potassium, sodium, zinc, phosphorus, magnesium, calcium, manganese; and is also loaded with chlorophyll. It's good for every part of your body – eyes, skin, nails, hair, heart, lungs, liver, and the list goes on. Start the day right, you never know what you may or may not eat later.

okay, so there are no peas in this recipe. but as John Lennon always told us "Give Peas a Chance!"

The Ultimate Veggie Breakfast Shake

This gorgeous, creamy, green veggie breakfast shake goes **one step further on the health-front** than The "Ultimate Fruit Breakfast Shake" (p. 95). The morning is without question the best time to get optimum liquid nutrition into your system. Your stomach is empty and the drink has a clear route through – which means it reaches the parts juices taken on a full stomach cannot get to.

Avocado
½ (ripe)

Golden Delicious Apples
2

Spinach
1 large handful

Courgette / Zucchini
3 cm chunk

Lime
1 (peeled)

Organic Carrots
2

Cucumber
¼ medium

Broccoli Stem
3 cm chunk

Celery
1 stalk

Green Bell Pepper
½

Ice Cubes
1 small handful

Make This Very Green Shake

Place one apple into the chute of the juicer (always making sure the juicer is 100% off) and then pack the spinach in tight behind it. Add the broccoli stem, lime, cucumber, pepper and courgette/zucchini and then sandwich with the other apple. Juice the lot then juice the stick of celery and carrots.

Place the ice and avocado into a blender and pour in the juice. Blend until smooth.

Start The Day With A Shake?

This veggie shake contains it all – the right essential fats, good quality proteins, the right carbs, vitamins, minerals, enzymes and organic water from within nature's finest water-rich foods. If you have this shake (and you eat three times a day) you have transformed one third of your diet to a 100% plant based vegan breakfast. Plus, despite the ingredients, it tastes amazing!

Mmm... Minerals!

As a rule of thumb vegetables are usually
mineral rich and fruits are vitamin rich.

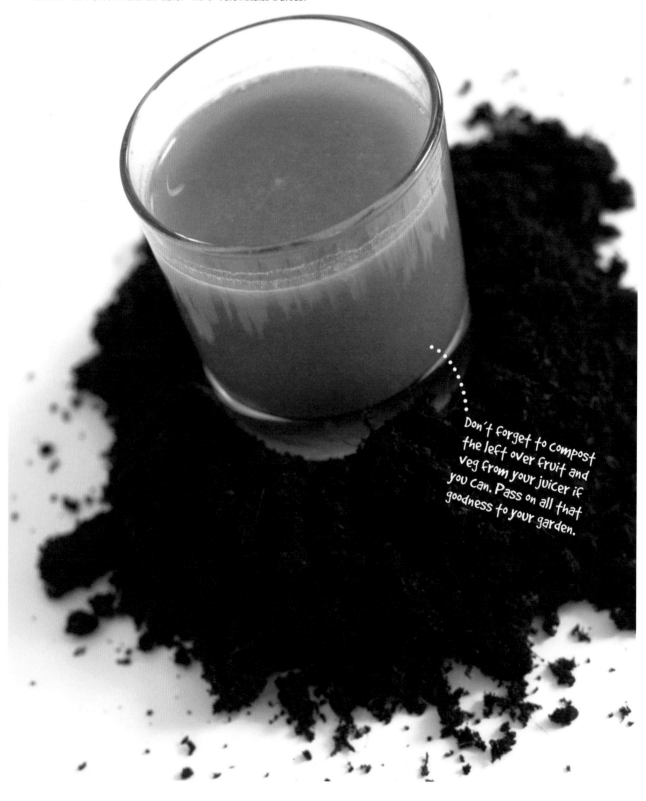

Don't forget to compost
the left over fruit and
veg from your juicer if
you can. Pass on all that
goodness to your garden.

Mineral Magic

Calcium, magnesium, phosphorous, zinc, potassium, sodium, copper, boron, manganese, sulphur, iron, chloride, selenium, and chromium are the big players in the mineral world. These are the ones we tend to recognize and the ones which many people are deficient in to a certain degree. However, there are, according to the science people, around 102 different minerals required by the human body for optimum health.

Golden Delicious Apples
2

Broccoli Stem
2 cm chunk

Spinach
1 large handful

Celery
½ stalk

Cucumber
¼ medium

Lime
½ (peeled)

Fresh Ginger Root
1 cm chunk

Ice Cubes
1 small handful

No Mining Required

Juice everything (except the wheatgrass) and pour over ice.

You can either make a wheatgrass shot separately and drink it just before or just after your main juice (if you do make sure you bite into a slice of orange just after the shot, as it tastes much better that way); or you can add a teaspoon of fresh wheatgrass powder to the whole drink and blend it up.

In order to make this super-mineral-rich, make *sure* you add the wheatgrass, but you can of course make the drink without.

Best Served... when you sense you are mineral deficient. Wounds not healing fast? Looking a little pale? Nails not growing? Losing your hair here and there? You can of course still have it if you are feeling perky, to prevent this from happening in the first place.

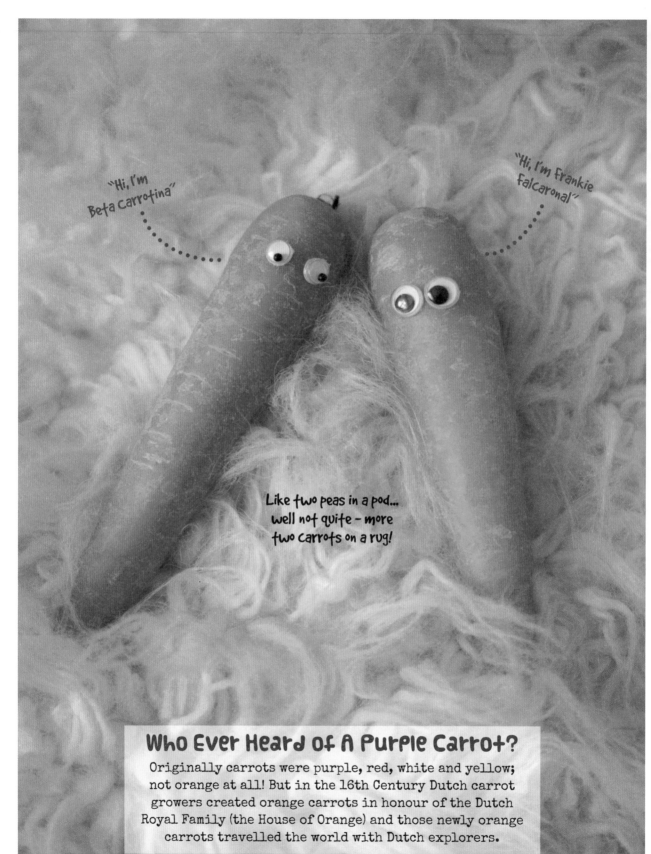

Who Ever Heard Of A Purple Carrot?

Originally carrots were purple, red, white and yellow; not orange at all! But in the 16th Century Dutch carrot growers created orange carrots in honour of the Dutch Royal Family (the House of Orange) and those newly orange carrots travelled the world with Dutch explorers.

Eye Love Carrots

There are some things in life which require a host of "bells and whistles" and others that just don't. It's like The Brits 2011 – so many performers with a whole host of special effects to enhance their performances; then on walked Adele, just her and a microphone: she totally stole the show!

It's the same for carrots, you can add all kinds of fruit 'n' veg, but the carrot is the undisputable king of simple juices. So here it is, carrots with a smidgeon of ginger. Do you **love carrots**?

Carrots
6 large

Fresh Ginger Root
3 cm chunk

Ice Cubes
1 small handful

How To Love Carrots

If you have only ever tasted carrot juice from a bottle, you are in for one heck of a treat!

It's so easy! Juice the carrots and ginger (as the optional supporting act) – no peeling required!

Pour over ice and enjoy.

Best Served... it's up to you where you'd like to have this juice.

All-Hail King Carrot

Carrots have everything! Vitamins A, B1, B2, B3, B6, C, E, and K. Minerals – potassium, iron, calcium, sodium, phosphorus, magnesium, silica, sulphur, chlorine and chromium. It's one of the best sources of beta-carotene (pro-vitamin A) on earth. Carrot juice is loaded with antioxidants and other nutritional goodies.

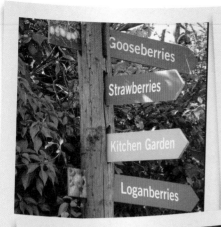

Gooseberries

Strawberries

Kitchen Garden

Loganberries

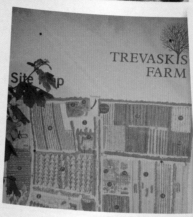

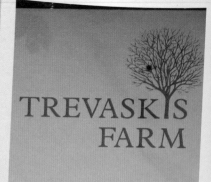

TREVASKIS
FARM

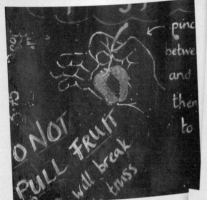

pinc
betwe
and
then
to

O NOT
PULL FRUIT
will break
truss

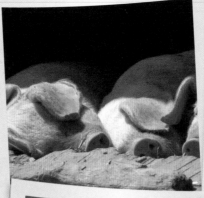

Site Map

TREVASKIS
FARM

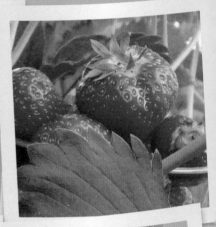

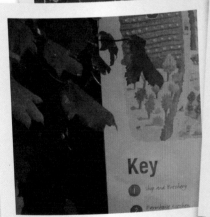

Key

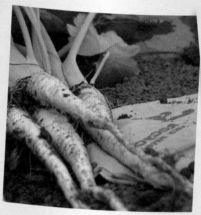

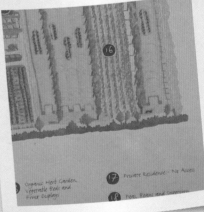

16

17

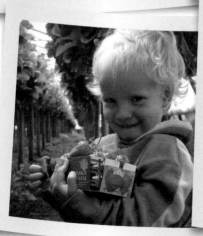

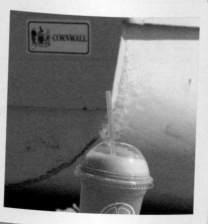

CORNWALL

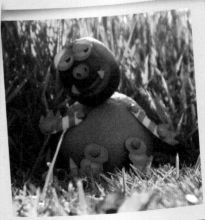

The Trevaskis Farm Smoothie

This recipe was created in honour of Trevaskis Farm. It's owned by a friend of ours, Giles, and he grows some of the finest produce I've ever tasted! In summer the farm is full of fresh strawberries, raspberries, loganberries, blackberries and blueberries all ripe and ready for you to pick yourself. The Trevaskis Farm smoothie is made from their **finest berries with a little extra fruit** from their trees.

Locally Grown Apples
2

Blackberries
1 small handful

Strawberries
1 small handful

Blueberries
1 small handful

Loganberries
1 small handful

Raspberries
1 small handful

Ice Cubes
1 small handful

Thanks For The Fruit Giles!

Juice the apples.

Place all the berries into the blender with the ice, add the apple juice and blend until smooth.

Best Served... at Trevaskis Farm with all the fruit, veggies and animals. It sits in gorgeous Cornwall countryside and is relatively close to some of the finest beaches in the world. I understand that if you are from London (as I originally was) you may not even be aware we have beaches in the UK but we do and Cornwall is famous for its golden sands and excellent surf. See "Cornish Lemon Surf" if you don't believe me.

If you're lucky enough to live near Hayle in Cornwall, pop in and get the ingredients from Giles at the farm.

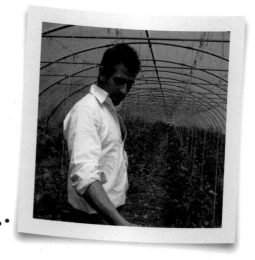

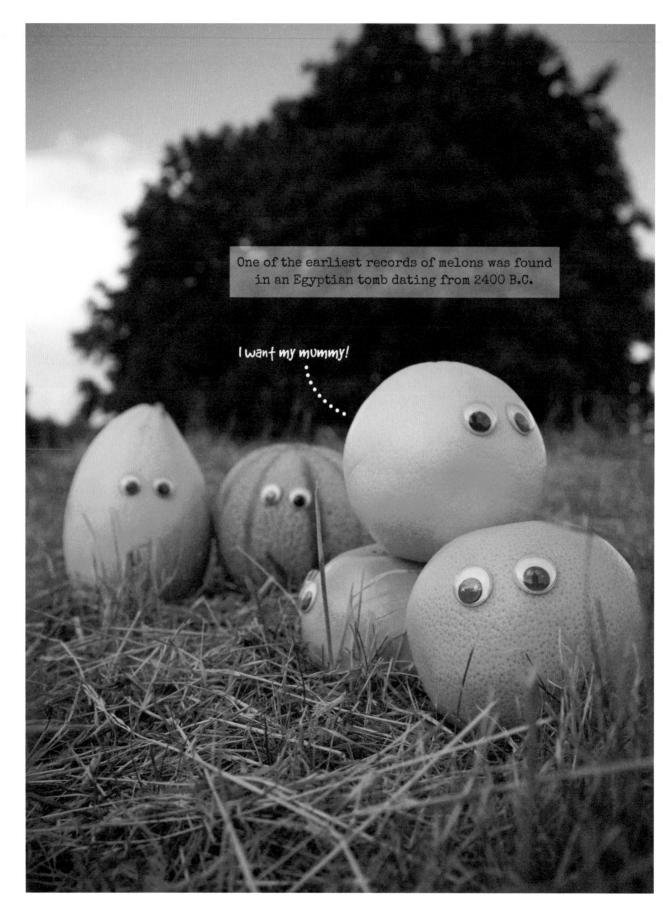

Honeydew Melon, Pineapple & Pink Grapefruit Crush

Some fruit juices taste good and some **take your taste buds to another place**. Honeydew Melon is one of those juices! It's gorgeous on its own, but with a little freshly extracted pineapple and pink grapefruit, it becomes simply heavenly.

Honeydew Melon
½ medium (flesh)

Pineapple
4 cm medium

Pink Grapefruit
½ medium (peeled)

Crushed Ice
I scoop

It's OK To Have A Little Crush

Pack the flesh of the melon tight into the chute of the juicer. Use the slowest speed to extract the most juice.

Peel the pink grapefruit, keeping as much of the white pith as you can.

Juice the pineapple (no need to peel if you have a good juicer) and grapefruit.

Pour in a glass over crushed ice.

Best Served… maybe in a bumblebee suit seeing as it's *Honey*dew melon. Or maybe not! Why not take this juice with you to the park and have it instead of an ice-cream?

More Than Just a Sweet Taste

Rich in vitamin C, potassium, pantothenic acid, and vitamin B6 which can help to combat high blood pressure, skin disorders and other related problems of the circulatory system.

When ripe, the Honeydew is the sweetest of all the melons. It's fat and cholesterol free and should be kept chilled – so store it in the fridge to keep it fresh.

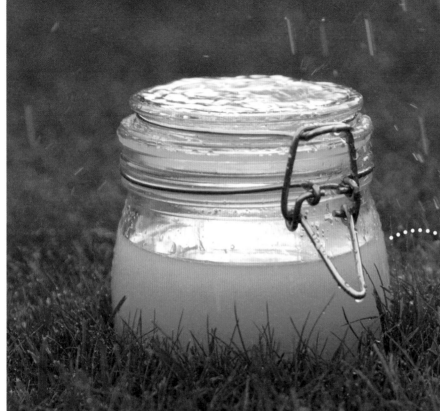

raindrops keep falling on my head!

Juicy Ginger Science

Ginger has fantastic anti-inflammatory properties. A
study in the "Journal of Medicinal Food" found that ginger
alleviated muscle pain more effectively than aspirin.

Broccoli, Ginger & Pineapple Punch

This simple combination packs a **powerful nutritional punch**. Sometimes "less is more" as they say, but what I always wondered is who *they* are? Hmmm… Enough of my meanderings, and on with the recipe!

Pineapple
¾ medium

Broccoli Stem
3 cm chunk

Fresh Ginger Root
2 cm chunk

Ice Cubes
1 small handful

Juicy Footsteps To Follow

Juice the pineapple (no need to peel if you have a good juicer), broccoli and ginger. Pour over the ice to make it refreshingly cool.

Best Served… this super little juice is just what you need if you're doing any physical work such as spending hours in the garden tending to the flowers or your veggie patch; or perhaps you've got a full weekend on with the kids; or you've got a day of shopping ahead and need the energy to get through trying on endless pairs of shoes. Me? I've been drinking them to give me the energy to write over 100 juice recipes!!

Broccoli Packs a Punch!

The little bonsai tree looking things that are broccoli are fantastic sources of vitamin C. A study at the University of South Carolina found that high doses of vitamin C (taken before and after exercise) reduce muscle soreness.

So this juice isn't just great for all you gym bunnies but also if you're doing any physical work

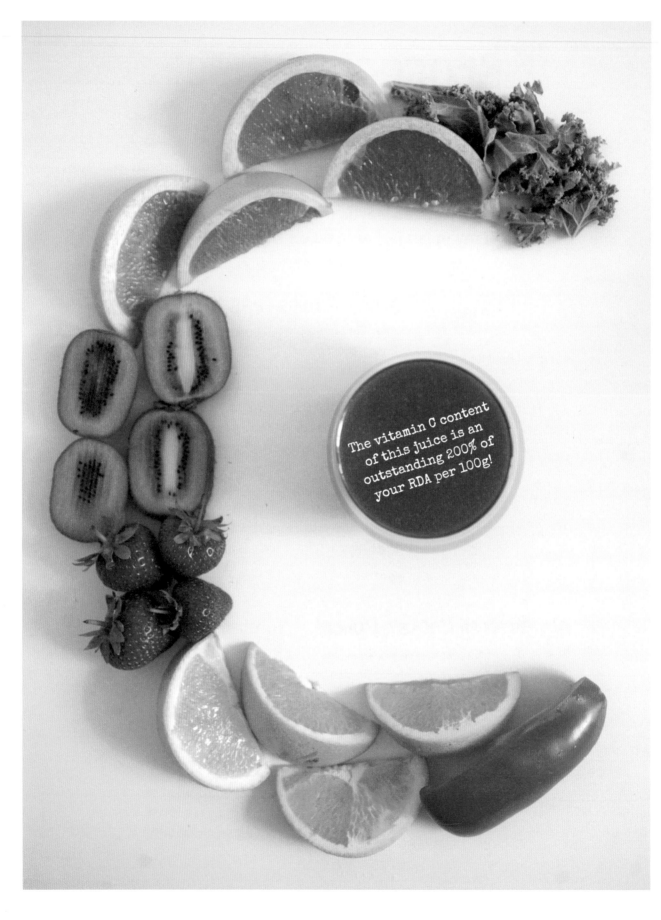

The vitamin C content of this juice is an outstanding 200% of your RDA per 100g!

Vitamin C Smoothie

This smoothie is bursting with ingredients that contain **high levels of vitamin C**. As you would expect you will find lots of gorgeous orange juice in this recipe but you will also find a few other ingredients that might surprise you...

"C" what I've done here?
oh never mind!

Oranges
2 (peeled)

Kiwifruit
1 (peeled)

Red Bell Pepper
¼

Grapefruit
1 medium (peeled)

Kale
1 handful

Strawberries
1 handful

Ice Cubes
1 small handful

"C" How To Make This Smoothie

Peel the oranges and grapefruit, keeping the white pith to make the juice more nutritious and creamier.

Juice the oranges, kiwi, pepper, grapefruit, and kale. Make sure you pack the ingredients tightly into the chute of the juicer to extract the most juice.

Pour the fresh juice into the blender, throw in a handful of strawberries, a small handful of ice and blend until smooth.

Best Served... to a friend or loved one who is perhaps a little poorly and needs a shot of vitamin C to get on the road to health.

What's So Important About Vitamin C?

Vitamin C is necessary for repairing and maintaining cells and bones as well as fighting infections, improving cholesterol, and it's thought to lower both cancer and cardiovascular disease risks.

Something that most people don't know however, is that the body cannot store vitamin C. It must continually be replenished through the diet, so have you topped-up your vitamin C levels yet today?

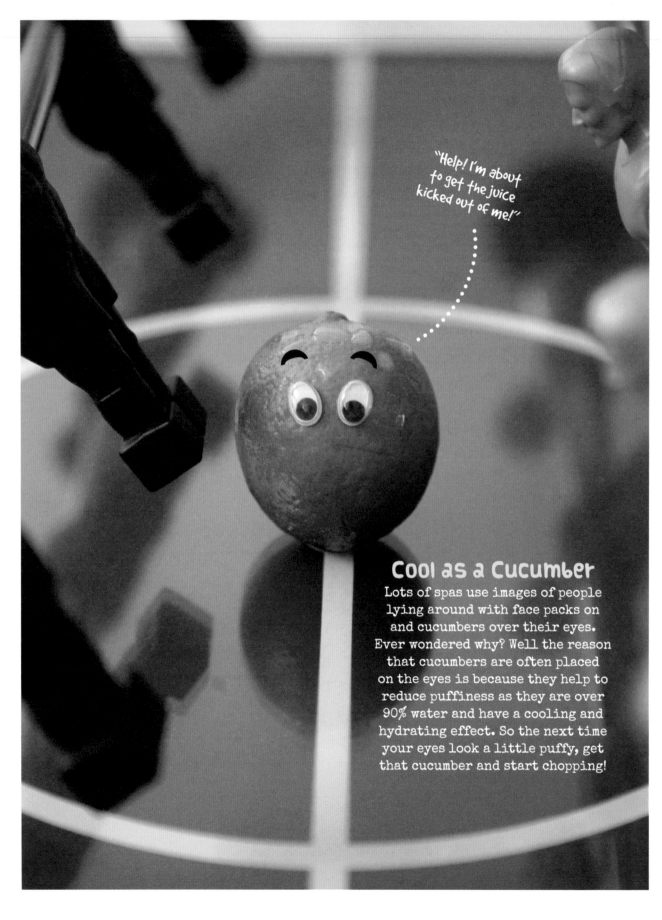

"Help! I'm about to get the juice kicked out of me!"

Cool as a Cucumber

Lots of spas use images of people lying around with face packs on and cucumbers over their eyes. Ever wondered why? Well the reason that cucumbers are often placed on the eyes is because they help to reduce puffiness as they are over 90% water and have a cooling and hydrating effect. So the next time your eyes look a little puffy, get that cucumber and start chopping!

Lime Green Smoothie

A delicate, creamy smoothie containing ripe avocado combined with the refreshing juices of an entire cucumber, a touch of spinach and spiced up with the **ultimate eastern taste combination** of lime and ginger.

Cucumber
1 medium

Lime
1 (peeled)

Fresh Ginger Root
2 cm chunk

Spinach
1 handful

Avocado
½ medium

Ice Cubes
1 small handful

Let's Kick-Off

Peel the lime, leaving as much of the white pith as you can.

Simply juice the cucumber, lime, ginger and spinach. Make sure you pack the spinach tightly into the chute of the juicer (before you start) to extract the most juice.

Pour the fresh juice into the blender. Add the ice and the avocado and blend until smooth.

Best Served... when your skin feels a little dehydrated. For optimum internal and external results, sit back in a chair drinking your smoothie through a straw with a couple of cucumber slices on your eyes.

Love cucumber – It Loves You!

Cucumber juice is really good for your hair, skin and nails. It's high in potassium and silica. Silica is important for healthy connective tissue, ligaments, cartilage, muscles, tendons, and bone.

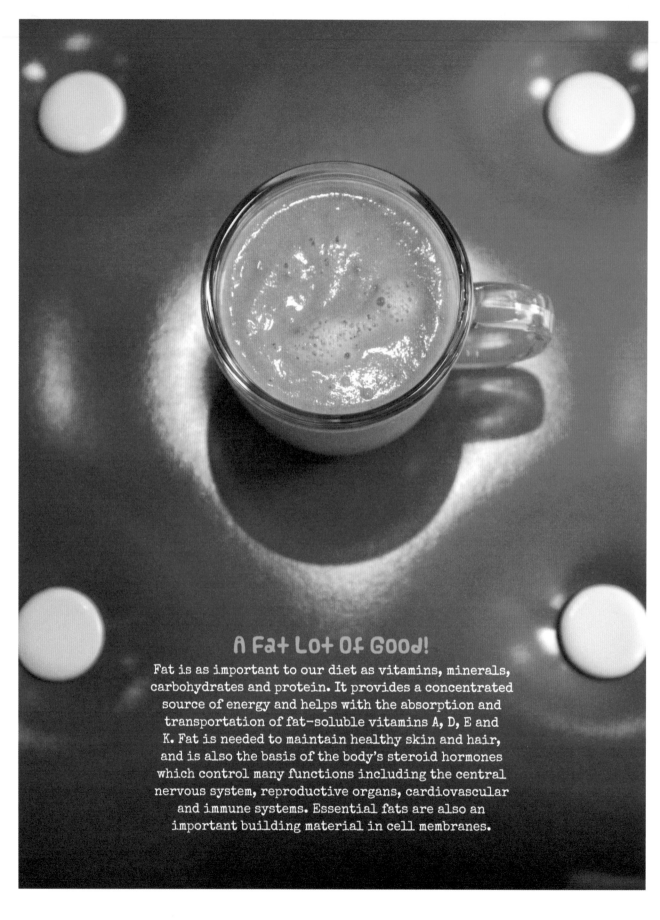

A Fat Lot Of Good!

Fat is as important to our diet as vitamins, minerals,
carbohydrates and protein. It provides a concentrated
source of energy and helps with the absorption and
transportation of fat-soluble vitamins A, D, E and
K. Fat is needed to maintain healthy skin and hair,
and is also the basis of the body's steroid hormones
which control many functions including the central
nervous system, reproductive organs, cardiovascular
and immune systems. Essential fats are also an
important building material in cell membranes.

The "EFA" Smoothie

If you're not familiar with the term "EFA" then I fully understand this might not sound like the most appealing recipe in this book. After all, an "Essential Fatty Acid" smoothie wouldn't quite get the same attention as a strawberry cream smoothie! However, (and this is a massive however) without EFAs your body simply wouldn't function as it should do, they're not called "essential" for the fun of it.

The good news is this recipe doesn't taste "fatty" or "acidy"... phew! In fact, it tastes **creamy, rich and surprisingly sweet**.

Pineapple
½ large

Kale
1 handful

Spinach
1 handful

Avocado
½ medium

Udo's Oil
1 heaped teaspoon
(or rape seed, hemp, or flaxseed oil)

Pumpkin Seeds (Pepita)
1 teaspoon

Sunflower Seeds
1 teaspoon

Walnuts
4 nuts (de-shelled)

Ice Cubes
1 small handful

"Essential" Instructions

Juice the pineapple (no need to peel if you have a good juicer), kale and spinach. Make sure you pack the greens tightly into the chute of the juicer, between the pineapple, to extract the maximum juice.

Pour the juice into the blender, add the remaining ingredients and blend until smooth.

Best Served... if the dark dog comes to visit, as a lack of EFAs has been associated with depression. So get blending and give your brain the good fats that it needs.

Not-So-Seedy

Sunflower seeds are not only rich in EFAs, they are also an excellent source of dietary fibre, amino-acids, vitamins and minerals.

Pumpkin seeds have been found helpful in preventing hardening of the arteries and have been used in the treatment of anxiety, depression and irritable bowel syndrome.

Eating 2-3 apricots will provide you with 50% of your daily value of vitamin A.

Apricots possess the highest levels and widest variety of carotenoids of any other food!

Astronauts ate apricots on the Apollo moon mission.

At Juicy HQ we believe that this smoothie will make you feel over the moon!

Apple, Mango & Apricot Medley

The flesh of ripe mango, torn from the stone, sits in perfect unison with the decadent juice of fresh apricots and delicate apples.

Be prepared for **something amazing** to happen!

Golden Delicious Apples
2

Fresh Apricots
4 medium (pitted)

Mango
½ medium (pitted & peeled)

Ice Cubes
1 small handful

How To Make This Medley

Remove the stone from the apricots.

Juice the apples and apricots. Make sure you pack the apricots tightly into the chute of the juicer, sandwiched between the apples, to get the most juice.

Carefully slice the mango just off-centre, avoiding the large stone inside, then scoop out the flesh from the skin into the blender. Add the freshly extracted juice and ice, and blend 'til smooth.

Best Served... when your taste buds are craving something new, something different, something sweet and something delicious!

What's Marvellous About This Medley?

This medley is like taking the most popular and least popular kids at school and teaming them up. Mangoes are one of the most commonly eaten tropical fruits. In contrast, apricots are often overlooked. Together they make a formidable partnership as an excellent source of vitamins A, C, E, dietary fibre, iron and potassium. Potassium is vital for maintaining pH levels in the body and regulating blood pressure.

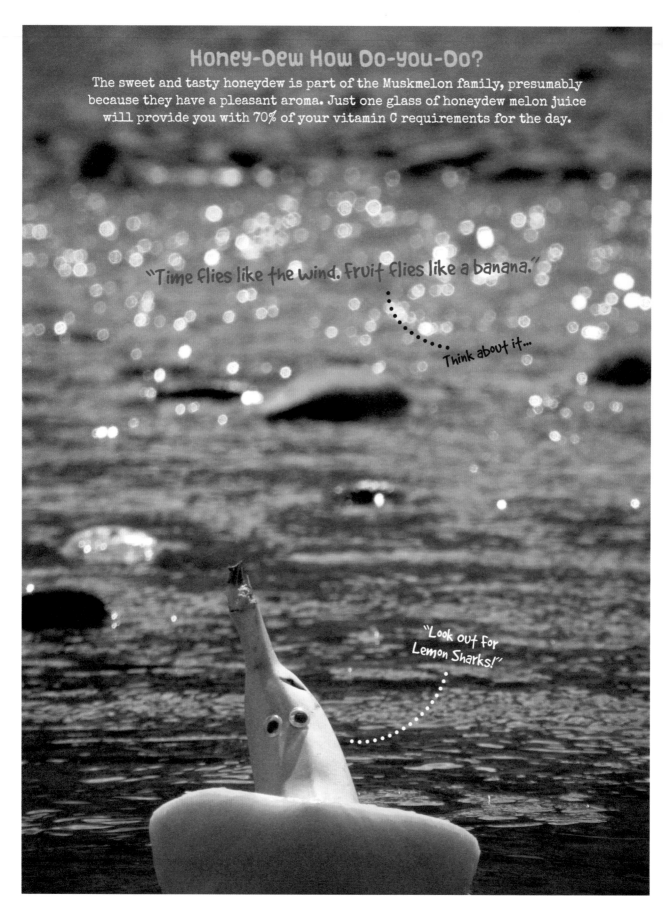

Melon Boat Bon-Voyage

Ideally melon is best drunk on its own, digestively speaking, but banana and honeydew go so stupidly well together on the taste front that this **gorgeous tasting smoothie** just had to go in the book.

Plus they look so good together!

Oranges
2 (peeled)

Banana
1 (ripe & peeled)

Honeydew Melon
½ small (seeded & peeled)

Cinnamon
a pinch

Ice
1 small handful

Sail Away on a Melon Boat

Peel the oranges, remembering to leave as much of the white pith as possible.

Juice the oranges and pour into the blender.

Scoop the flesh from the melon into the blender, along with the peeled banana, and ice. Blend until gorgeous.

Pour in a cool glass and sprinkle on the cinnamon, it makes this already lovely smoothie even scrummier.

Best Served... lying on a boat made from half a honeydew melon whilst pretending to be a banana. Or first thing in the morning, wherever you are.

Don't Wander off!

Did you know that the banana "tree" is not really a tree, it's actually a giant herb; and it can "walk" up to 15 cm a year!

Stringy Bits

Don't complain about those stringy bits in bananas, they're called "pholem bundles" and they help to transport the nutrients to all parts of the fruit.

ain Entrance ↑

ll Wards & Departments) →

est Entrance ↑

ight Access) ↑

Suffering from an emergency health situation?
Follow this sign and get to the hospital asap! →

Suffering from a common aliment or the first signs of ill health? Maybe
you can avoid this place altogether with a little juicy help from Dr Juice! ←

rth Entrance

Centre →

Dr Juice

"Let Juice Be Thy Medicine"

I'm Not A "Real" Doctor - Glad That's Clear!

Over the years I have seen just about every common ailment either improve or completely disappear with the help of freshly extracted juice. This, I believe, is because every single fruit and vegetable designed for human consumption was designed by nature to feed and heal the body. "Natural Juice Therapy" works so well for so many different conditions because the life-giving nutrients contained within all nature's foods are extremely easy for the body to ingest and utilize in juice form. Unlike conventional drug therapy, juice therapy rarely, if ever, has any adverse side-effects; and because the pure nutrient filled liquid was designed by nature, it treats the body as a whole and doesn't try to heal selectively. This is why so many "different" ailments are helped with juicing.

Once the body gets what it needs to strengthen the immune system, everything gets better.

However, despite instinctively knowing this, we live in a world of pharmaceutical influence and the vast majority of us seek drug-therapy as our first point of call to help disease; not our desperate last-ditch attempt to cure our ills once nature has appeared to have failed.

The Only Serious Bit Of The Book

What many are unaware of is the potential danger of pumping our systems with medical drugs week after week. In 2006 over 1 million people in the UK were admitted to hospital because of the adverse drug reactions from the pharmaceutical drugs they were prescribed. These people took the drugs as they were directed to. The cost to the British taxpayer was £2 billion. In 2009 1.2 million people needed emergency treatment because they "abused" the medical drugs they were given – an increase from 627,000 in 2004. If you combine the adverse drug reactions from people taking the drugs "as directed" and the people abusing medical drugs:

You have over 2 million people a year in hospital because of medical drugs.

These are the same drugs which have apparently been developed to save them!

It is also worth knowing perhaps that in the US 140,000 people die each year from adverse drug events and another 88,000 die from acquired infections in hospital, making a total of 228,000 deaths a year. This makes it the third leading cause of death in the United States – only behind heart disease and cancer according to the CDC's statistics.

Every day 640 people and each week 4,384 people are dying from adverse drug reactions or hospital acquired infections. That's nearly 10% of all deaths – or more than a World Trade Centre attack every week.

The War on Disease

The medical industry put these deaths down to "collateral damage" and in the war on disease there will be some casualties. However, if Natural Juice Therapy caused over 100,000 deaths per week in one country alone, do you think I would be allowed to continue practicing? Actually if Natural Juice Therapy killed just one person it would be front page news and the medical industry would want me in prison. Okay! Rant over!

This may sound as though I am totally against drug based medicine – *I am not.* I used to suffer from severe asthma and without my asthma pump I genuinely don't believe I would be here today. Short-term medical intervention is absolutely necessary in certain circumstances. But that's the problem: not only are we becoming a nation that rattles as it walks, we seem oblivious to the adverse side-effects or how long we have been popping the same pills and potions.

A Refreshing Approach

For those who are willing to expand their mind and look a little further than the pill for every ill doctrine, there is another way. In this section I have picked 15 of the most common ailments and have designed different combinations of freshly extracted juices and smoothies to help the body heal and treat itself. When I was a boy and cut or grazed my knee, as long as I left it alone, it would heal itself. You will see on wildlife programmes how, when primates break a bone, there are times when it will mend itself. The body will heal, if it's given the chance and has the right nutrients to help with the repair. Although you may not see your condition here, it doesn't mean juicing will not help. You need to understand that two things usually cause most common ailments and disease and treatment for most is the same.

Toxicity & Deficiency

If you remove the "toxicity" and replace the "deficiencies" the body usually finds its balance and equilibrium of natural health. In other words, if you stop flooding your body with rubbish foods and drinks and furnish it with the finest liquid fuel containing all of the essential vitamins, minerals, amino acids, carbohydrates, essential fatty acids, enzymes, and co-factors – 90% of ailments seem to improve or go away completely. However, there are certain natural substances in certain fruits and vegetables which can help specific conditions; I mentioned there are 15 here.

I must point out at this stage that *I am not a doctor* and so I have to say: "please consult your family doctor before using anything other than medical drugs to treat your condition". Yes it is mad, but that's the world we live in. You need to seek medical approval in order to use nature's plants to heal your body – "Go figure!" as they say in the good ol' U.S. of A.

Please make sure that if you are on any medical drugs *whatsoever* for any condition, consult your doctor before coming off them. There are also certain juices which prevent certain medical drugs from working, so please, *please* make sure you do your home-work and ask your doctor **first** before using Natural Juice Therapy to treat any aliment.

I Sincerely Hope The Juicy Lifestyle Works For You

Make a point of reading some of the stories in the "Community Juice" section (p. 120) or read some of the life-changing stories on my website. If you do see a change for the better, please drop me a quick email and who knows you may find yourself in the next book.

If you need further help please contact one of the Independent Juice Master Trained Natural Juice Therapists (see www.juicemaster.com).

MEMORY & RECALL

ASTHMA

BLOOD PRESSURE

CHOLESTEROL

PSORIASIS, ECZEMA & ACNE

HANGOVERS

ANAEMIA

HAY FEVER

PREGNANCY

DIABETES

HEALTHY BONES

COLDS & FLU

SLIMMING

ARTHRITIS, CRAMP & GOUT

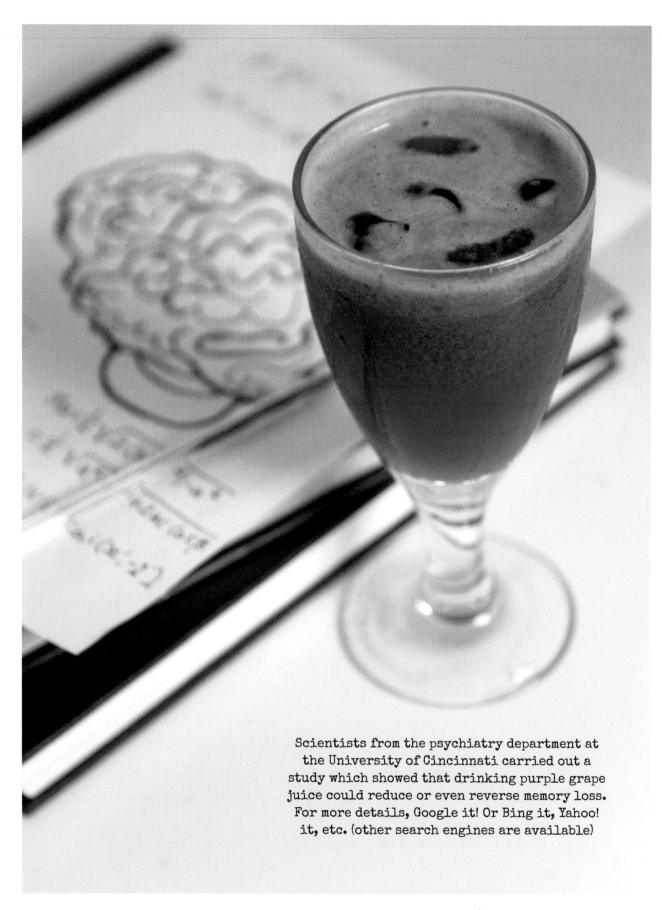

Scientists from the psychiatry department at the University of Cincinnati carried out a study which showed that drinking purple grape juice could reduce or even reverse memory loss. For more details, Google it! Or Bing it, Yahoo! it, etc. (other search engines are available)

Total Recall
The Memory-Aid Juice

PRESCRIPTION
FOLLOW DIRECTIONS BELOW
TO BE TAKEN AS REQUIRED

JHS
Juicy Health Service

Apples
TWO GOLDEN DELICIOUS

Purple or Red Grapes
ONE LARGE HANDFUL

Blueberries
ONE LARGE HANDFUL

Ice Cubes
ONE SMALL HANDFUL

INSTRUCTIONS: Pack the grapes and blueberries tightly into the chute of the juicer, behind one of the apples, followed by the other apple on top. Juice slowly to ensure you get the maximum amount of juice out of the grapes and blueberries.
Serve over ice and sip slowly like a fine wine.

BEST SERVED: when you need to keep your memory in peak condition.

A study was conducted a few years ago which concluded that if you drink juice three times a week you are 75% less likely to get Alzheimer's Disease. Personally I don't feel the study took into account as many variables as it should and I am not 100% convinced of its validity. However, there is strong evidence that apples help the brain to increase production of an essential chemical.

fresh apple juice maintains levels of the neurotransmitter acetylcholine

Acetylcholine is vital for memory and brain health, and low levels are linked to Alzheimer's. Add this to the studies done on grape and blueberry juice and you may find you soon won't have to look up this recipe, you'll remember what's in it!

Breaking News

A study conducted at the Center for Cellular Neurobiology and Neurodegeneration Research at the University of Massachusetts Lowell, showed that apple juice could help Alzheimer's disease. The study showed that mice receiving the human equivalent of two glasses of apple juice a day for a period of 1 month produced lesser amounts of the beta-amyloid protein. This protein is believed to be the culprit behind the formation of "senile plaques", which are most commonly found in patients suffering from Alzheimer's Disease.

Head of the research, Dr. Shea, states that "These findings provide further evidence linking nutritional and genetic risk factors for age-related neurodegeneration and suggest that regular consumption of apple juice can not only help to keep one's mind functioning at its best, but may also be able to delay key aspects of Alzheimer's disease..."

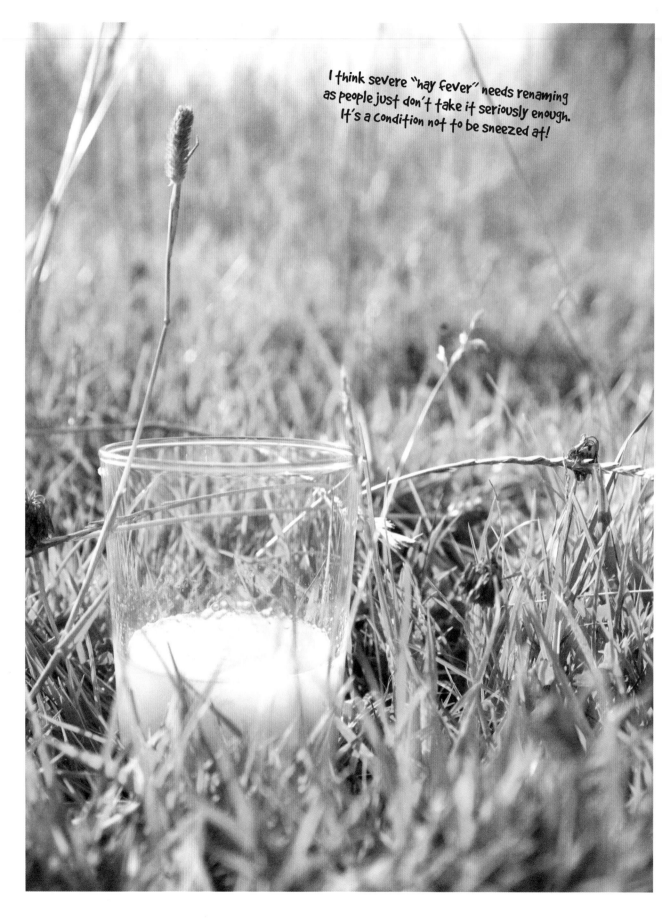

I think severe "hay fever" needs renaming as people just don't take it seriously enough. It's a condition not to be sneezed at!

Hay Fever Heaven
The Anti-Histamine Super Shot

PRESCRIPTION
FOLLOW DIRECTIONS BELOW
TO BE TAKEN AS REQUIRED

JHS
Juicy Health Service

Ginger Root
6 cm CHUNK

Lemon
HALF UNWAXED

Apple
ONE LARGE

Ice Cubes
ONE SMALL HANDFUL

```
------------------------------------------------
INSTRUCTIONS: Simply juice the lot.
------------------------------------------------
BEST SERVED: every single morning for at
least four weeks BEFORE your pollen season
starts. Then every day during the whole
season.
Best taken in a small "shot" glass and downed
in one.
I wish you a tissue, tablet and nasal spray
free summer.
------------------------------------------------
```

This was another ailment I used to suffer from in a bad way. Like many diseases, there is a spectrum of severity for this particular disease. For some, hay fever means slightly itchy eyes and a bit of a sniffle; for others it means feeling like you have been run over by a truck. I was in the "run over by a truck" hay fever camp.

I HAD to find either an air-conditioned building or a sauna to get any respite at all!

I really wish they would rename this "Severe Hay Fever" as people just don't take hay fever seriously. If you do suffer badly, my heart goes out to you. Even more so if every year you find you have to pump your body full of drugs. The good news is that there is a natural remedy, which actually seems to work and I would like to present it to you here. I am not saying it will 100% clear all of your symptoms but there is no harm in giving it a go as unlike most drugs, it's "adverse side-effect free" (unless you are allergic to the ingredients of course!) It works for me every year and I hope it will work for you.

"Dear Jason,
I have suffered from terrible hay fever for many years – blocked nose, sneezing, generally feeling awful. I came across one of your books half-way through this year's hay fever season, within 2 days symptoms had completely gone. Then the only way I was aware that the hay fever season had ended was when my hay fever suffering colleagues at work (who had foolishly not taken my advice to use the book) told me that their symptoms had finally gone. Definitely the most effective health book I have ever read!"

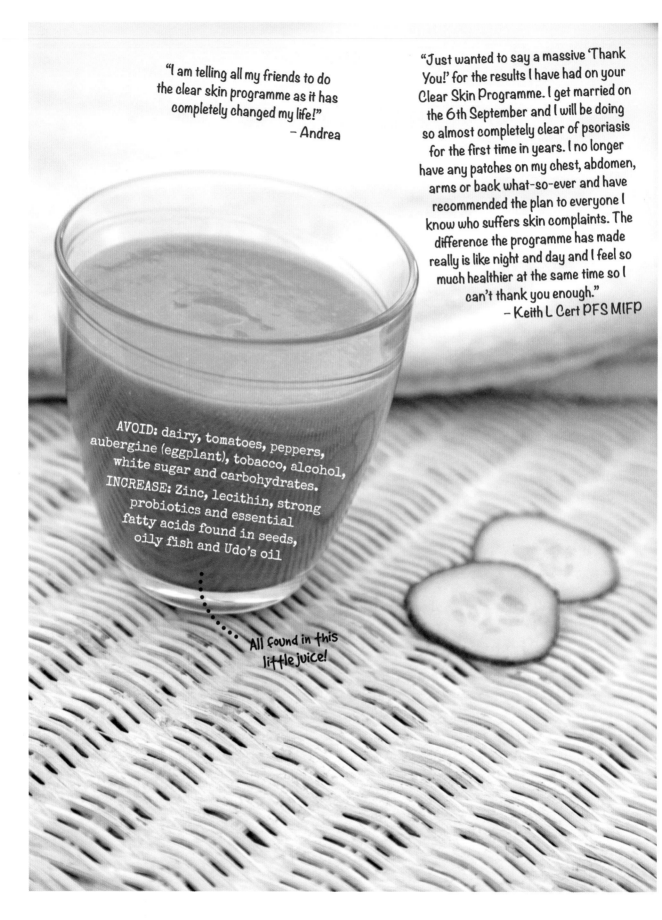

"I am telling all my friends to do the clear skin programme as it has completely changed my life!"
– Andrea

"Just wanted to say a massive 'Thank You!' for the results I have had on your Clear Skin Programme. I get married on the 6th September and I will be doing so almost completely clear of psoriasis for the first time in years. I no longer have any patches on my chest, abdomen, arms or back what-so-ever and have recommended the plan to everyone I know who suffers skin complaints. The difference the programme has made really is like night and day and I feel so much healthier at the same time so I can't thank you enough."
– Keith L Cert PFS MIFP

AVOID: dairy, tomatoes, peppers, aubergine (eggplant), tobacco, alcohol, white sugar and carbohydrates.
INCREASE: Zinc, lecithin, strong probiotics and essential fatty acids found in seeds, oily fish and Udo's oil

All found in this little juice!

Clear Skin Smoothie
The One For Psoriasis, Eczema & Acne

PRESCRIPTION
FOLLOW DIRECTIONS BELOW
TO BE TAKEN AS REQUIRED

JHS
Juicy Health Service

Apples
TWO GOLDEN DELICIOUS
Pineapple
3 cm SLICE
Fresh Ginger Root
2 cm CHUNK
Lemon
ONE-THIRD
Cucumber
ONE-QUARTER MEDIUM
Avocado
ONE-HALF (RIPE)
Mixed Seeds
ONE TABLESPOON
Lecithin Granules
ONE HEAPED TEASPOON
Udo's Oil
TWO TEASPOONS

INSTRUCTIONS:
Juice the apples, pineapple, ginger, lemon and cucumber.
Put the avocado, seeds, lecithin granules and oil into the blender. Add the juice, a little ice and blend until smooth.

BEST SERVED: if you have psoriasis this is best served at the Dead Sea. If you have the chance go there for at least two weeks (preferably four), lie down for as long as possible. You will come back tanned and your skin will be amazing. And if you have fresh fruit like zinc-rich watermelon every day with this smoothie — that's even better. If you can't get to Israel, best served at home on an empty stomach.

Having suffered from severe psoriasis and eczema myself for many years and having cleared myself of both conditions through diet change, I feel I am somewhat qualified to write on this subject.

Every inch of my body was covered in psoriasis

Firstly my heart goes out to you if you have any skin condition and particularly if you have a severe case of one. In my case virtually every inch of body was covered in psoriasis (including my face) and the backs of my knees had bad eczema. It can affect every single part of your life. I have put together a 64 page "Clear Skin" **free** download. Go to www.juicemaster.com, where will see a "free downloads" button. This has all the information you need in terms of exactly what to consume and, moreover,

what to avoid. For now, if you don't want to follow a strict programme but simply want something that may improve your skin, then this smoothie has the perfect nutrition for the job. I wish to make something clear however, I am not suggesting this "Clear Skin" super smoothie alone will clear you of whatever skin condition you have.

This one Smoothie Alone will not cure you, but it should help to a great extent.

There are many contributing factors that make up psoriasis, eczema and acne and this one smoothie alone will not "cure" you. However, it should help to a great extent if you replace your breakfast every day with this smoothie. That way you have instantly turned one third of what you consume per day into a 100% plant based meal.

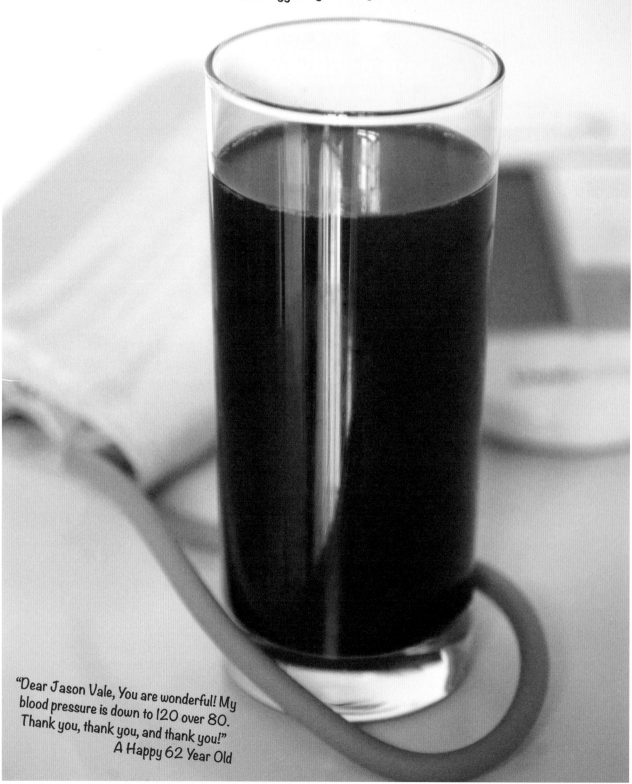

"Dear Jason, I had to go to the doctors on Monday and they took my blood pressure... it was normal! When I first went on your juicing retreat I was taking tablets for high blood pressure and I am so pleased that I was able to come off them (something my doctor said would not happen). I have kept off them ever since by juicing. Thank you".

"Dear Jason Vale, You are wonderful! My blood pressure is down to 120 over 80. Thank you, thank you, and thank you!"
A Happy 62 Year Old

Ease The Pressure
A Natural Way To Lower Blood Pressure

PRESCRIPTION
FOLLOW DIRECTIONS BELOW
TO BE TAKEN AS REQUIRED

JHS
Juicy Health Service

Raw Beetroot
3 SMALL BULBS

Apples
TWO GOLDEN DELICIOUS

Grapes
BLACK OR RED
1 LARGE HANDFUL

Ice Cubes
ONE SMALL HANDFUL

INSTRUCTIONS: Simply juice the lot, pour over ice and enjoy.
When juicing grapes don't forget to pack them in the juicer tight to get the most juice (making sure your machine is off when you pack them down!)

BEST SERVED: if you've just got an unjust parking ticket from a warden who is on commission (how did that ever happen?!) or you've been eating all the pies…

Here is a simple, effective and scientifically proven way to lower your blood pressure using only the power of the juice. Nuff said!

Blood Pressure Science Report

A daily glass of red grape juice may help men with hypertension lower their blood pressure, according to results from a preliminary study presented in the US in 2003.

In the study, men with raised blood pressure who drank Concord grape juice for 12 weeks experienced a significant drop in both their systolic and diastolic blood pressures.

Latest Beetroot News!

Researchers at Barts and The London School of Medicine have discovered that drinking just 500 ml of beetroot juice a day can significantly reduce blood pressure. Professor Ahluwalia and her team found that in healthy volunteers, blood pressure was reduced within just 1 hour of ingesting beetroot juice, with a peak drop occurring 3-4 hours after ingestion. Some degree of reduction continued to be observed until up to 24 hours after ingestion. Researchers showed that the decrease in blood pressure was due to the chemical formation of nitrite from the dietary nitrate in the juice.

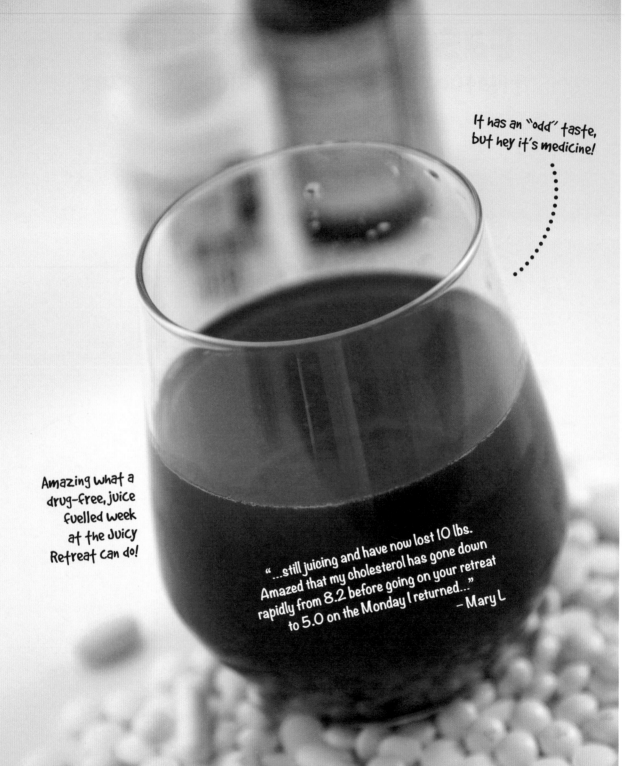

It has an "odd" taste, but hey it's medicine!

Amazing what a drug-free, juice fuelled week at the Juicy Retreat can do!

" ...still juicing and have now lost 10 lbs. Amazed that my cholesterol has gone down rapidly from 8.2 before going on your retreat to 5.0 on the Monday I returned..."
– Mary L

"My cholesterol level has dropped down to 6.2 and then 4.7 from 6.9 within the first few weeks of juicing and over time I am now down to 3.9! The doctor is astonished at these results and claims that "even medication would not have got it down to this level and in such quick time"
– Wayne

The Cholester-Low
The Natural Statin

PRESCRIPTION
FOLLOW DIRECTIONS BELOW
TO BE TAKEN AS REQUIRED

JHS
Juicy Health Service

Black Grapes
ONE SMALL HANDFUL

Red Grapes
ONE SMALL HANDFUL

Apple
TWO GOLDEN DELICIOUS

Fresh Ginger Root
3 cm CHUNK

Raw Beetroot
ONE BULB

Vine-Ripe Tomato
ONE SMALL

INSTRUCTIONS: Pack the grapes tightly into the chute of the juicer behind one of the apples. Add the ginger, raw beetroot and tomato, and sandwich the lot between the other apple. Juice on the slow setting and push through slowly.
Pour over ice and drink slowly.

BEST SERVED: in hospital to help people in recovery. The last time I went into a hospital I simply heard the "ping" of a microwave going off. It's odd that most people end up in hospital because of the wrong foods, and once there they still can't get any decent food!

Welcome to the new holy grail of the pharmaceutical industry – cholesterol lowering drugs, or statins as they are known. Statins are the single biggest drug cost to the NHS and such is the desire by Big Pharma to get everybody taking these drugs it was even suggested statins be put in our drinking water!

The Cholesterol "Con"!

May I suggest you read *The Cholesterol Con* by Malcolm Kendrick. It may just shed some light on what I believe to be one of the 21st Century's biggest medical hoodwinks. If you are taking statins consult your doctor before coming off them; however, I have a ton of emails from people who have reduced their cholesterol simply by removing the junk and adding some juice. What may surprise you is that it is still not agreed by all in the medical field that elevated cholesterol levels cause heart disease, or in fact exactly what high cholesterol even is. It changes from decade-to-decade and *Big Pharma* know that if they move the "healthy" cholesterol level from say 6 down to 5, they've just captured another million people who overnight now have "dangerous" levels of cholesterol. This way they get to sell many millions more drugs – simples!

There are now over 1 million prescriptions for statins every week in the UK

When you think all drugs have degrees of adverse side effects, that's a frightening number. However, if you are worried for whatever reason about your cholesterol levels, start your juicing lifestyle with this juice, remove the "crap" from your diet, jump on a treadmill and allow your body to find its natural cholesterol level – whatever your body deems that to be.

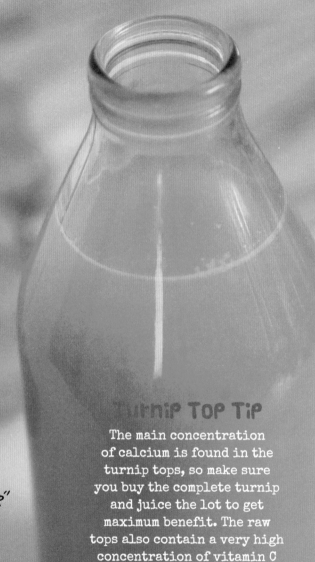

Turnip Top Tip

The main concentration
of calcium is found in the
turnip tops, so make sure
you buy the complete turnip
and juice the lot to get
maximum benefit. The raw
tops also contain a very high
concentration of vitamin C
(twice as much as oranges),
as well as vitamins B, E and
beta-carotene. They also
contain the minerals iron,
phosphorus and potassium.

That's a "turnip"
for the books

The Bone Builder
The Calcium King

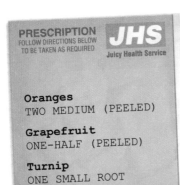

Oranges
TWO MEDIUM (PEELED)

Grapefruit
ONE-HALF (PEELED)

Turnip
ONE SMALL ROOT

Carrot
ONE LARGE

Ice Cubes
ONE SMALL HANDFUL

INSTRUCTIONS: Peel the oranges and grapefruit (leaving as much of the white pith as possible). Juice the lot, pour over ice and drink slowly.

BEST SERVED: as often as possible if you suffer from osteoporosis. Also best served after a long walk, a good run, doing some weights, or any physical activity which will all help "dem bones", "dem bones"... etc. :)

It appears the belief that the best way to build our bones is by consuming as many dairy foods as possible isn't going away, if anything it's getting stronger... unlike our bones! The fact we are the only creatures on earth who still drink milk after weaning age doesn't appear to dissuade the vast majority of people from this strongly held belief.

Even Cows Don't Drink Milk!

However, it is not so much a case of where you are getting your calcium from more, what is robbing you of it. Soft drinks, coffee, refined sugar and so on, are all acidic and leach calcium from the bones. The biggest irony I guess is that pasteurised cow's milk is acidic once ingested by a human, meaning it can actually cause the body to leach calcium in certain circumstances. With this in mind I would first advise you to skip so many acid-forming foods and get this

beautiful calcium rich alkaline juice inside your body. It will give the body a chance to build the bones at least – plus it's another juice with science on its side:

Orange & Grapefruit Juice Builds Bones In Rats!

A team at Texas A&M, conducted a study which showed rats fed orange and grapefruit juice had improved bone density. After examining the bones at the cellular level, they found that a reduction in bone density is caused when there is an increase in oxidants. In these studies, both grapefruit juice and orange juice increased antioxidants in the rats' systems. So that is the benefit since oxidants damage bone cells... "There are about 400 compounds in citrus," the team reported. "So we need to find out which compound in citrus caused this." I don't think you need find out "which" compound is the magic one. Common sense should tell us that nature works synergistically and it's the combination of all its nutrient factors which help every aspect of health – in this case the building of bone density.

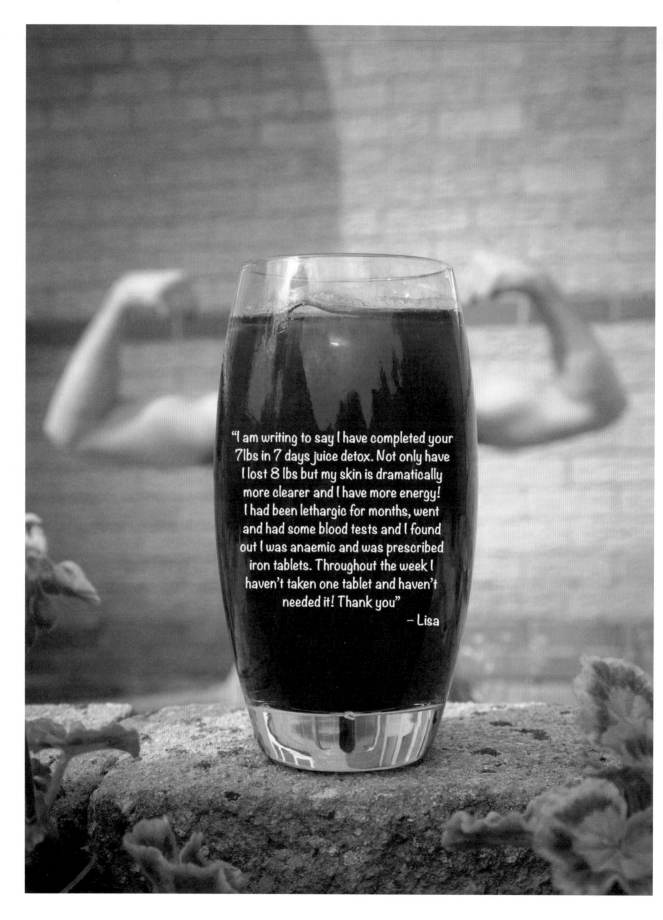

"I am writing to say I have completed your 7lbs in 7 days juice detox. Not only have I lost 8 lbs but my skin is dramatically more clearer and I have more energy! I had been lethargic for months, went and had some blood tests and I found out I was anaemic and was prescribed iron tablets. Throughout the week I haven't taken one tablet and haven't needed it! Thank you"

– Lisa

Yes this works just as well for women, but "Iron Man" is better as a title!

Iron Man
The One For Anaemia & Iron Deficiencies

PRESCRIPTION
FOLLOW DIRECTIONS BELOW
TO BE TAKEN AS REQUIRED

JHS
Juicy Health Service

Kale
ONE LARGE HANDFUL
Spinach
ONE LARGE HANDFUL
Apples
TWO GOLDEN DELICIOUS
Broccoli Stem
3 cm CHUNK
Raw Beetroot
ONE SMALL BULB
Green Bell Pepper
ONE HALF (SEEDED)
Ice Cubes
ONE SMALL HANDFUL
Wheatgrass
ONE "SHOT" PLUS
SEGMENT OF ORANGE

INSTRUCTIONS: Pack the kale and spinach tightly into the chute of the juicer behind one of the apples. Add the broccoli, beetroot, bell pepper (remove the seeds) and close with the last apple. Juice the lot and pour over ice if you want to cool it down. The idea is to have your wheatgrass shot as a chaser (i.e. after the juice). Because the wheatgrass isn't to everyone's taste, you should drink the shot in one hit and take a bit of a piece of orange immediately afterwards.

BEST SERVED: when one is feeling a little pale!

Anaemia is a decrease in number of red blood cells or less than the normal quantity of haemoglobin in the bloodstream. Anaemia is the most common disorder of the blood and, although there are many kinds, the most common can be treated with a good dose of iron.

A Great Blood Builder!

This juice has an extremely high iron content, making it a great blood builder. This concoction regenerates and reactivates the red blood cells and supplies fresh oxygen to the body. Please note this "Iron Man" juice works well without the wheatgrass if you really cannot get hold of any, but the wheatgrass takes it to another level for the treatment of anaemia – I highly recommend you get some if you suffer badly from this condition.

Hot Iron News

One cup of spinach juice contains 377% of your RDA for vitamin A, 84% of your magnesium requirements, 65% of your daily folate needs and 35% of your iron requirements. Red beet juice is associated with human blood and blood forming qualities. Due to its higher content of iron, it regenerates and reactivates the red blood cells, supplies fresh oxygen to the body and helps the normal function of vesicular breathing (i.e. normal breath sound). It is therefore extremely useful in the treatment of anaemia. Broccoli juice is an excellent blood purifier and cleanser and contains plenty of iron. Kale juice is also an amazing source of easy to assimilate iron and the green pepper has been added as it's extremely high in vitamin C. Vitamin C aids the body's ability to absorb iron. For all the benefits of Wheatgrass juice see page 254

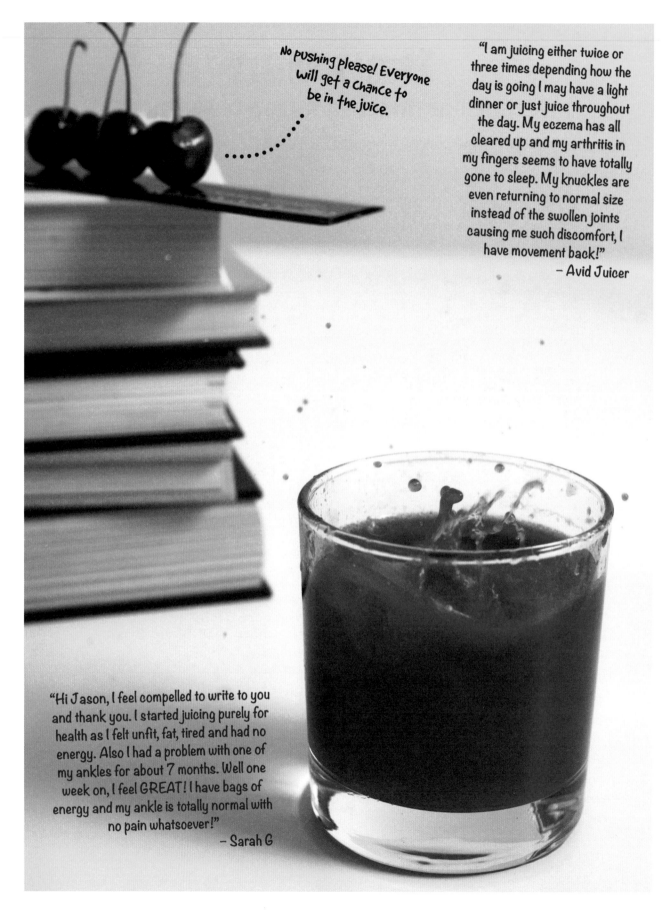

Arthritic Elixir
Easy relief for Arthritis, Cramp & Even Gout

PRESCRIPTION
FOLLOW DIRECTIONS BELOW
TO BE TAKEN AS REQUIRED

JHS
Juicy Health Service

Pineapple
ONE-QUARTER MEDIUM

Cherries
ONE LARGE HANDFUL
(PITTED)

Celery
2 STALKS

Grapefruit
ONE-HALF MEDIUM
(PEELED)

Ice Cubes
ONE SMALL HANDFUL

INSTRUCTIONS: Pack the cherries (with the pits removed) tightly into the chute of the juicer followed by the grapefruit (peeled — but with as much white pith left on as possible), pineapple (no need to peel if your juicer will take it) and celery. Juice the lot, pour over ice and enjoy.
If you find you are not a grapefruit person — as many people aren't — simply make the juice without the grapefruit but with a whole medium pineapple.

BEST SERVED: when your joints are feeling a little stiff, or better still before - prevention is always king!

Over the years I have seen some quite incredible things happen with many aliments, none more so than with stiff joints. I have seen people come to our retreat unable to walk properly due to severe arthritis and, within seven days of juicing, climb a small mountain (no, this is not an exaggeration).

I have seen people unable to bend their fingers gain full movement within just a week.

If you do suffer from arthritis, please remove ALL dairy foods, ALL white refined sugars and carbohydrates and wheat products while at the same time drink the following juice twice a day. As always make sure you tell your physician first and do not come off any medical drugs until you get permission from your lovely doctor. I sincerely hope you get some respite from this often incredibly debilitating condition.

Read All About It!

In 1950 a study in Texas proved just how effective cherry juice can be for gout and arthritis. Twelve gout suffers were given the equivalent of 1lb of cherries or the equivalent amount of cherry juice. What they found was in every case uric acid levels went down to normal and they didn't suffer any more attacks of gouty arthritis. That's every single case!

Pineapple juice is one of the only sources of the strong anti-inflammatory enzyme bromelain. Bromelain helps the body to break down protein. Incomplete protein breakdown (i.e. poor digestion) is a condition implicated in arthritis.

The polyacetylene in celery juice is perfect for the relief for all inflammation including rheumatoid arthritis, osteoarthritis, gout, asthma and bronchitis.

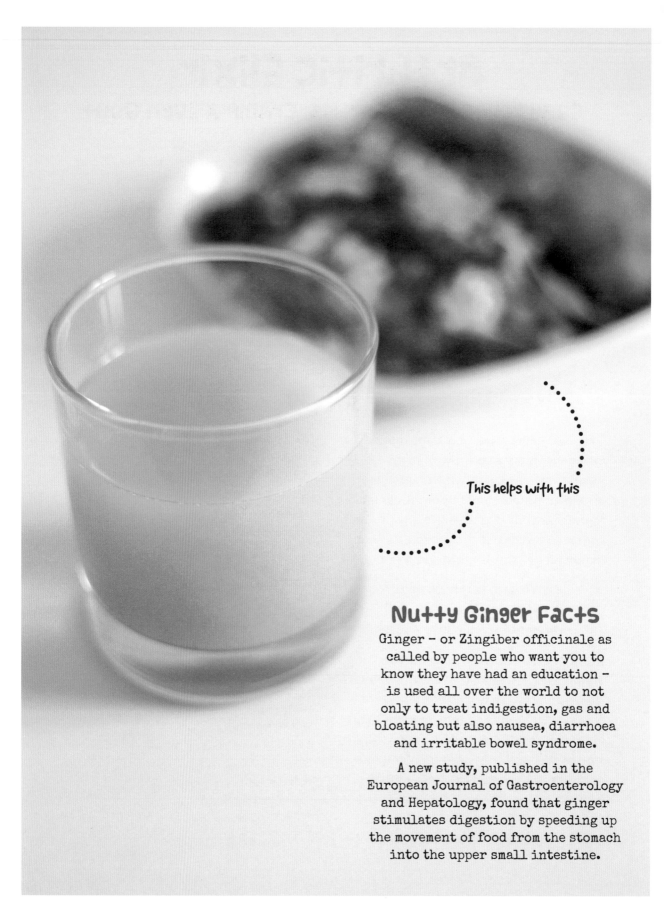

This helps with this

Nutty Ginger Facts

Ginger – or Zingiber officinale as called by people who want you to know they have had an education – is used all over the world to not only to treat indigestion, gas and bloating but also nausea, diarrhoea and irritable bowel syndrome.

A new study, published in the European Journal of Gastroenterology and Hepatology, found that ginger stimulates digestion by speeding up the movement of food from the stomach into the upper small intestine.

Digestive Aid
The One for Your Digestive System & Indigestion

PRESCRIPTION
FOLLOW DIRECTIONS BELOW
TO BE TAKEN AS REQUIRED

JHS
Juicy Health Service

Pineapple
3 cm SLICE (PEELED)

Fresh Ginger Root
2 cm CHUNK

Fennel
2 cm CHUNK

Lemon
ONE-THIRD MEDIUM

Pear
ONE-HALF MEDIUM

Fresh Mint
ONE SMALL HANDFUL

INSTRUCTIONS: Juice everything except the mint.
You can either pour the juice into a blender, add the mint and blend. Or to save having to wash the blender, you can simply chop the mint very finely, add to the juice and stir.

BEST SERVED: sipped slowly throughout your meal to "aid digestion", or drunk just before you eat. If you only require a small shot (as you may not want the juice to spoil your hunger) simply leave out the pear and use a smaller slice of pineapple — it will still do the trick. If you have problems digesting protein always leave the pineapple in.

The easiest way to solve digestion problems for most people is to stop eating 'foods' which the body has difficulty digesting. I am sure we are the only creatures on earth who need an antacid! **All** fruits and vegetables have been virtually predigested by the plant and require very little work from us to digest, extract the nutrients, and dispose of the waste.

Go With Your Gut Instinct!

However, if you do suffer from digestive issues try this natural Digestive Aid, it may help, it may not – but with no adverse side-effects and nothing but goodness, it won't do you any harm. I would recommend sipping throughout your meal or having all of it just before you eat. If your digestive issues continue I would highly recommend taking some quality digestive enzymes and friendly bacteria with your meal.

Pear is rich in vitamins C and B1 and has diuretic and anti-bacterial effects. FYI: It is also useful for kidney stones and urinary infections.

Lemon Juice helps the stomach's digestive ability by adding to the digestive juices and acid. Some people cannot completely digest their food before it is released into the intestine – sometimes called "leaky gut". The liver sees them as contaminants – food particles, even tiny ones should not be in the bloodstream. The liver filters them out which improves the digestion process relieving the liver of the filtering load.

Mint promotes digestion and soothes the stomach in cases of indigestion and inflammation. The aroma of mint activates the saliva glands in our mouth as well as glands which secrete digestive enzymes, thereby facilitating and helping digestion.

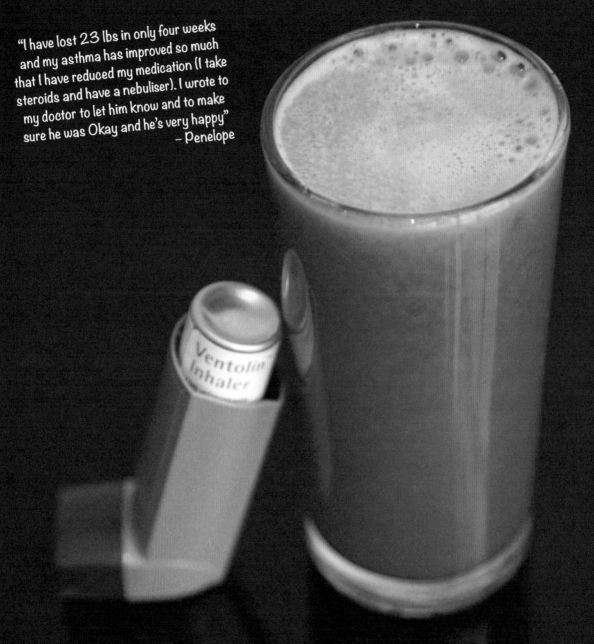

"I have lost 23 lbs in only four weeks and my asthma has improved so much that I have reduced my medication (I take steroids and have a nebuliser). I wrote to my doctor to let him know and to make sure he was Okay and he's very happy"
– Penelope

The Juicy Science Bit

The National Heart and Lung Institute research, published in the European Respiratory Journal: Children who drank apple juice at least once a day were half as likely to suffer from wheezing as those drinking it less than once a month. Interestingly, the study also concluded that eating fresh apples themselves gave no apparent benefits, leading the researchers to conclude the juice must be more bio-available. Dr Peter Burney, who led the project, said that it was possible that 'phytochemicals' in apples, such as flavonoids and phenolic acids, were helping to calm the inflammation in the airways which is a key feature of both wheezing and asthma.

Asthma Tonic
The One To Help You Breathe A Little Easier

PRESCRIPTION
FOLLOW DIRECTIONS BELOW
TO BE TAKEN AS REQUIRED

JHS
Juicy Health Service

Apples
TWO GOLDEN DELICIOUS

Pineapple
ONE-QUARTER MEDIUM
(PEELED)

Celery
TWO STALKS

Fresh Ginger Root
3 cm CHUNK

Raspberries
ONE SMALL HANDFUL

Ice Cubes
ONE SMALL HANDFUL

INSTRUCTIONS: Juice the apples, pineapple, celery and ginger.
Pour the juice into the blender, add the raspberries and ice then blend.

BEST SERVED: on an empty stomach and drink at least twice a day for noticeable results.

EXTRA TIP: Avoid all dairy food; white refined sugar and carbohydrates as well as wheat. For a two week period also avoid all from the deadly nightshade family — bell peppers, tobacco, aubergine (eggplant) and tomatoes as many with asthma find that these aggravate their condition.

I had my first asthma attack when I was eight years old. I was given the blue inhaler immediately and progressed rapidly to the brown (steroid) one. I would have to have at least one inhaler with me at all times - just the realization of being without one would send me into an attack. I used the blue one around 14-16 times a day, every day. I was told there wasn't a cure and, like with my psoriasis, it was never even suggested diet could play a part at all.

My Asthma Completely Vanished

Since changing my diet and massively increasing my fresh fruit and vegetable intake through the power of juicing, my asthma has vanished. I am not suggesting that your asthma will be cured by simply drinking this juice, but I know of many people for whom a change of diet and the incorporation of fresh juices has helped tre-mendously. I am also aware of many people who have indeed managed to stop using their inhalers. I wish to make extremely clear that you should never stop using your inhaler without seeing your doctor first. I sincerely hope you get some degree of help from this juice and the little tips.

"I am 32 years of age and have been a severe asthmatic since the age of seven. Since following your plan I no longer have to reach for the inhaler 3 times a day. It's so wonderful to wake up in the morning without broken sleep as I am dreaming or trying to find my pump as I am wheezing in my sleep."
– Laura

"Thanks for inspiring my life with juice. 8 months straight now! And my girlfriend too - and she has dropped her asthma spray. What more can you ask for?"

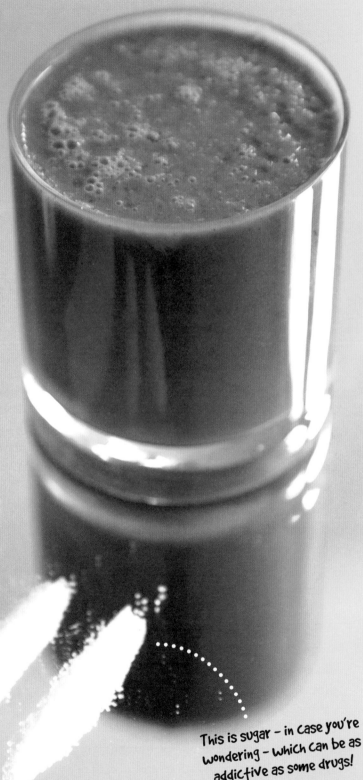

"...because of one of your books I bought a juicer and have become a juicing addict shedding those excess pounds with ease in the process. Best of all the hypoglycaemia which has plagued me for over 10 years is under control and I have far more energy and stamina... many, many thanks"
– Kay

This is sugar – in case you're wondering – which can be as addictive as some drugs!

Diabetes Aid
A Balancing Act For Insulin Production

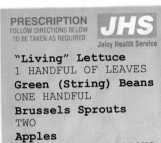

PRESCRIPTION
FOLLOW DIRECTIONS BELOW
TO BE TAKEN AS REQUIRED

JHS
Juicy Health Service

"Living" Lettuce
1 HANDFUL OF LEAVES

Green (String) Beans
ONE HANDFUL

Brussels Sprouts
TWO

Apples
TWO GOLDEN DELICIOUS

Carrots
TWO MEDIUM

Avocado
ONE-HALF RIPE
(PEELED)

Cinnamon
TWO HEAPED TEASPOONS

Ice Cubes
ONE SMALL HANDFUL

INSTRUCTIONS: "Living Lettuce" is quite new to most supermarkets. It's the lettuce you can buy that is still growing inside little pots of mud — because of this they are incredibly fresh.
Pack the lettuce, string beans and brussels sprouts tight into the chute of the juicer behind one of the apples; put the other apple on the top. Juice these ingredients and then juice the carrots.
Pour the juice into a blender then add the avocado, cinnamon and ice. Blend to perfection.

You may be reading this with surprise – a juice suitable for treating diabetes! It's widely believed that juices and diabetes don't mix due to how quickly the sugars are released into the bloodstream. However, having observed people with diabetes on our retreats (where we consume nothing but fresh juices) I can safely say freshly extracted juices drunk slowly and slightly watered down have no adverse effect with type 2 diabetes. That said, although this is what I have observed from the retreats and from the many emails I have received – this is not scientific. Always consult your doctor.

Freshly extracted juices are not the same as "cooked" juices.

From everything I have observed over the years I am of the belief that freshly extracted juices do not give the same spike in blood sugar as cooked juices.

The smoothie I have created here contains avocado. This beautiful fruit is loaded with good fats and fibre, both of which help to slow down the absorption of sugars in the bloodstream.

Rid Your Pancreas of Excess Fat

If the pancreas is full of fat it stands to reason that it won't be able to pump insulin effectively. When someone rids themselves of excess fat, insulin can once again be released and blood sugar returned to normal. So as well as this smoothie, I would highly recommend reducing your intake of "crap" foods, especially white refined sugars and carbohydrates, whilst at the same time increasing your exercise. This smoothie alone will not reverse diabetes, but if you swap one of your meals for this smoothie, you have transformed a third of your diet in one easy swoop. Happy Days! *PTo...*

THERE ARE NOW 3 MILLION PEOPLE IN THE UK WITH DIABETES AND RISING BY 17 PEOPLE EVERY HOUR!

THE COST TO THE NHS IS 3.5 BILLION POUNDS AND RISING EVERY SECOND!

GLOBALLY 285 MILLION PEOPLE HAVE THE CONDITION RISING TO AN ESTIMATED 438 MILLION BY 2030!

THERE ARE MORE AMPUTATIONS DUE TO DIABETES THAN THERE ARE BECAUSE OF SMOKING!

CINNAMON CAN SIGNIFICANTLY INCREASE YOUR GLUCOSE METABOLISM WHICH IMPROVES BLOOD SUGAR REGULATION. JUST HALF A TEASPOON OF CINNAMON PER DAY HAS BEEN FOUND TO SUBSTANTIALLY REDUCE BLOOD SUGAR LEVELS.

CINNAMON HAS BEEN FOUND TO HAVE "INSULIN-LIKE EFFECTS" DUE TO A BIO-ACTIVE COMPOUND, QUALIFYING IT AS A CANDIDATE FOR AN INSULIN SUBSTITUTE.

CINNAMON SLOWS THE EMPTYING OF YOUR STOMACH TO REDUCE SHARP RISES IN BLOOD SUGAR FOLLOWING MEALS, AND IMPROVES THE EFFECTIVENESS, OR SENSITIVITY, OF INSULIN.

News Just In

Researchers at Newcastle University conducted a study in 2011 where 11 men and women with type 2 diabetes were put on a diet of 600 calories a day for 8 weeks. After just one week, some of their blood sugar readings had returned to normal. After two months, fat levels in the pancreas had returned to normal and the organ was able to pump out insulin without any problems. That's **EVERY SINGLE ONE OF THEM**. Lead author, Professor Roy Taylor said, "This is a radical change in our understanding of type 2 diabetes. While it has long been believed that the disease will steadily get worse, we have shown that we can reverse it"

A STUDY PUBLISHED IN 2009 STATED, "POLYPHENOLS FROM CINNAMON COULD BE OF SPECIAL INTEREST IN PEOPLE WHO ARE OVERWEIGHT WITH IMPAIRED FASTING GLUCOSE, SINCE THEY MIGHT ACT AS BOTH INSULIN SENSITIZERS AND ANTIOXIDANTS."

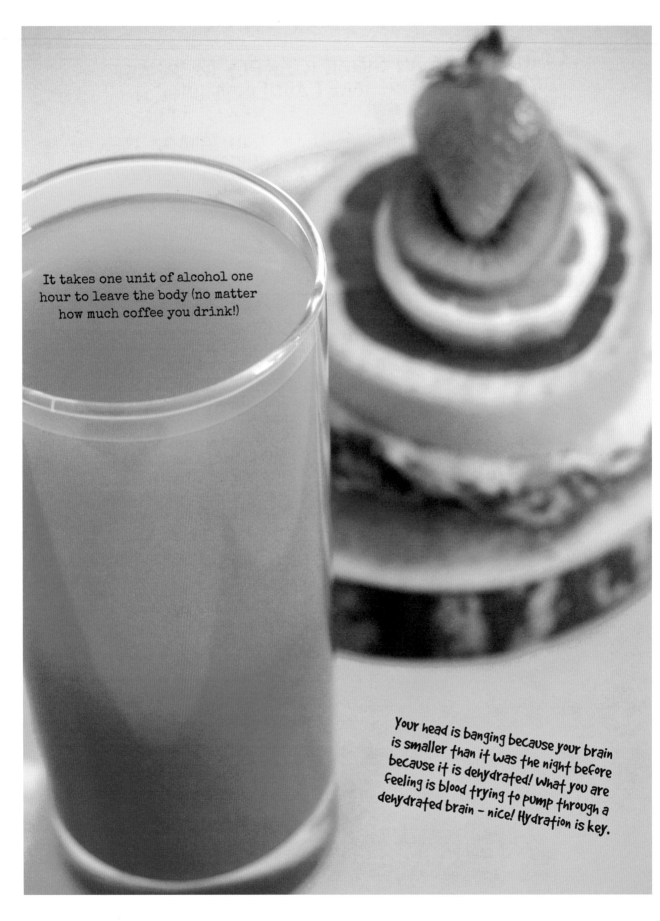

It takes one unit of alcohol one hour to leave the body (no matter how much coffee you drink!)

Your head is banging because your brain is smaller than it was the night before because it is dehydrated! What you are feeling is blood trying to pump through a dehydrated brain – nice! Hydration is key.

Hangover Helper
For the Grizzly Bear In Your Head

PRESCRIPTION
FOLLOW DIRECTIONS BELOW
TO BE TAKEN AS REQUIRED

JHS
Juicy Health Service

Watermelon
ONE QUARTER MEDIUM (PEELED)
Kiwifruit
ONE (PEELED)
Pink Grapefruit
ONE-HALF (PEELED)
Pineapple
ONE-HALF MEDIUM (PEELED)
Lime
ONE-HALF
Strawberries
ONE HANDFUL
Ice Cubes
ONE SMALL HANDFUL

INSTRUCTIONS: Juice the Watermelon, kiwifruit, grapefruit, pineapple and lime and pour into a blender along with the strawberries and ice and blend.

BEST SERVED: in bed, reading the Sunday papers before taking the dog for a walk.

The best way to avoid a hangover is perhaps an obvious one – don't drink! Okay, a tad facetious I am sure you'll agree. So if you do drink and have perhaps overdone it, this will do the trick. This smoothie contains ultra-hydrating watermelon, vitamin B3 rich kiwifruit, metabolism boosting grapefruit, powerful protein digesting pineapple, vitamin C packed lime and antioxidant rich strawberries. All of which should sort your head and body out!

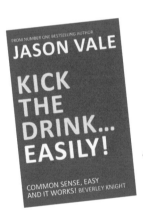

FROM NUMBER ONE BESTSELLING AUTHOR
JASON VALE
KICK THE DRINK... EASILY!
COMMON SENSE, EASY AND IT WORKS! BEVERLEY KNIGHT

If you're having more than an occasional tipple, this might come in handy!

Pre Hangover Tip

If you are going to drink you need to understand that you tend to drink one pint and pee out three! With this in mind drink one alcoholic drink followed by a glass of water and repeat if you fancy getting squiffy. Before bed, drink about ½ litre of water – it makes all the difference to how your head feels the next day.

"I am well impressed. And I have booted booze out of my life and don't miss it! I never thought I would be free of the booze craving, but now have no fear of not drinking. Excellent read. Jason really is a life-saver!"

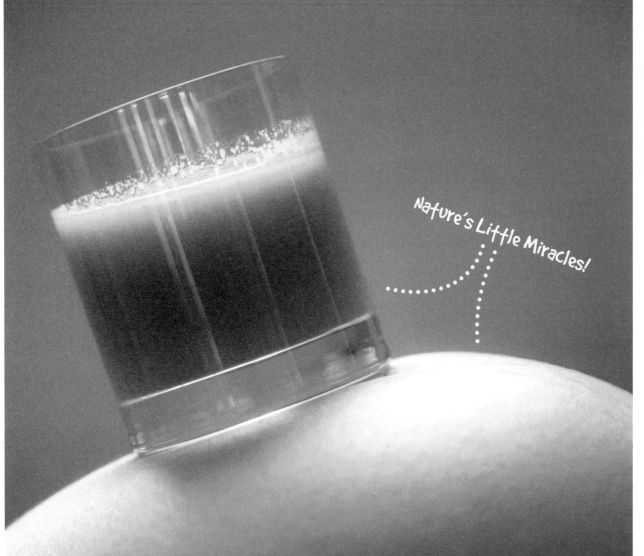

Nature's Little Miracles!

A little factoid about this smoothie for you to pass on to the little one in a few years

Sunflower seeds are a high source of folic acid, protein, some of the B vitamins, vitamin E and many minerals, such as iron, magnesium, calcium and selenium. 100g of sunflower seed kernels contain 227 µg of folic acid, about 37% of the recommended daily intake. So now you know! Oh and the little ones might also like to know that asparagus is a nutrient-dense food which again is high in folic acid and is a good source of potassium, fibre, vitamin B6, vitamins A and C, and thiamine. Avocado was in the Guinness book of records as "the most nutritious fruit on earth", it's loaded with vitamin E. Vitamin E is an antioxidant supplement that contains natural tocopherol, which helps support your brain, and cardiovascular and respiratory systems; peace of mind when feeding your "bun in the oven".

Bun In The Oven
For A Healthier Pregnancy

PRESCRIPTION
FOLLOW DIRECTIONS BELOW
TO BE TAKEN AS REQUIRED

JHS
Juicy Health Service

Spinach
1 SMALL HANDFUL
Pineapple
ONE-QUARTER MEDIUM
(PEELED)
Asparagus
4 SPEARS
Apple
ONE GOLDEN DELICIOUS
Fresh Peas
ONE HANDFUL
Sunflower Seeds
ONE SMALL HANDFUL
Avocado
ONE-HALF RIPE
(PEELED)
Ice Cubes
ONE SMALL HANDFUL

INSTRUCTIONS: Before you turn on the juicer
put the apple into the juicer chute. Then
pack the peas, spinach and asparagus in tight
and add the pineapple in chunks.
Juice the lot slowly to get maximum juice.
Put the sunflower seeds into the blender along
with the ice and avocado. Blend until smooth.

BEST SERVED: while standing in the
beautifully decorated room that awaits the
most precious thing you will ever have in
your life. Sip while you take in the enormity
of the situation, and enjoy your "meal for
two".

There is so much conflicting advice about what mothers-to-be should be eating. It appears to change on a weekly basis.

Expecting mothers require the finest nutrition available

One piece of advice, which rarely changes and is generally agreed across the board, is that mothers need the best nutrition possible. It is also widely agreed that good quality fruits and vegetables contain essential vitamins, minerals, carbohydrates, essential fats, organic rich water, enzymes and other co-factors yet to be truly identified, which are vital for mother and baby. As it's the juice contained within the fibres that provide these nutrients, fresh juicing is a perfect way for those with a "bun in the oven" to feed the cells of mother and baby. It's also worth knowing that virtually all fruit and vegetables contain folic acid, essential for expecting mothers. A lack of folic acid can lead to a folate deficiency which can result in many health problems, the most notable one being neural tube defects in developing embryos. This "Bun In The Oven" juice contains an abundance of folic acid, hence the peas and asparagus (they are in for a good reason!) as well as many other vital nutrients. As always, you need to consult your doctor, but just on an instinctive level, it just makes sense.

"Hello Jason, not only was the juice diet very successful and I lost the desired amount, but I also got pregnant whilst juicing! We were so happy as I had been having problems getting pregnant. Anyway, we are now proud parents of little Sophie who is 4 weeks old and I just wanted to share this success story with you!"
– Nicola

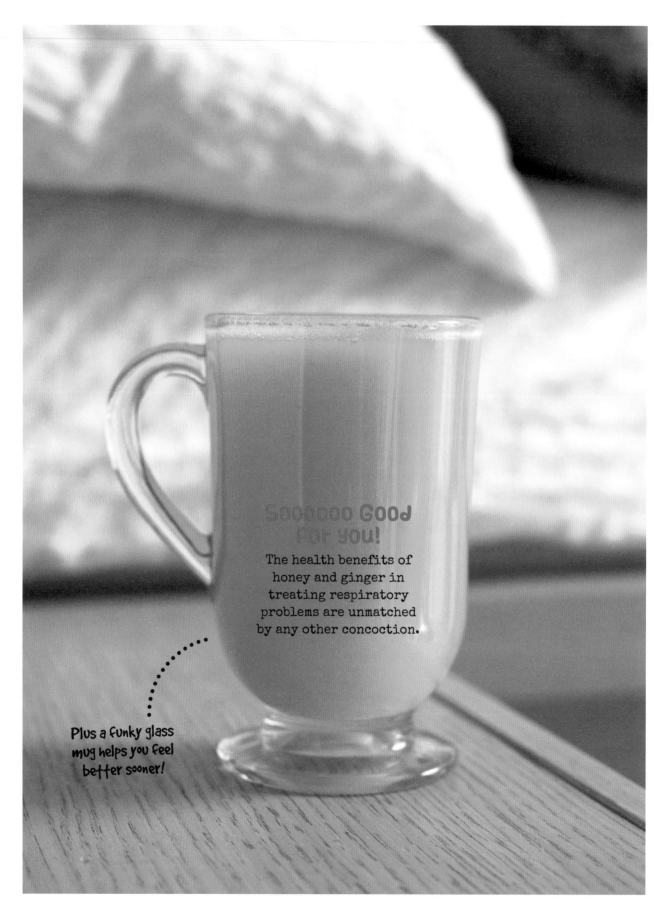

Sooooooo Good
For you!

The health benefits of
honey and ginger in
treating respiratory
problems are unmatched
by any other concoction.

Plus a funky glass
mug helps you feel
better sooner!

J'M-SiP
For Colds & Flu - It's A Hottie!

PRESCRIPTION
FOLLOW DIRECTIONS BELOW
TO BE TAKEN AS REQUIRED

JHS
Juicy Health Service

Apple
ONE GOLDEN DELICIOUS

Fresh Ginger Root
3 CM CHUNK

Lemon
ONE-HALF (UNWAXED)

Manuka Honey
ONE HEAPED TEASPOON

Hot Water
ONE HALF CUP

INSTRUCTIONS: Juice the apple, ginger and lemon (leave the peel on).
Pour the juice into your favourite mug. Make sure you only half fill the mug and then top up with hot (not boiling) water from the kettle.
Add the Manuka honey, stir well and sip your way back to health.

BEST SERVED: If you need one of these, chances are you are lying in bed watching Jeremy Kyle, tissues by your side. This should soon have you up on your feet!

This is the Juice Master's take on a Lemsip, only without a drug in sight. It has become widely known as the J'M-sip (pronounced "Jemsip"). Fresh apple, ginger and lemon juice mixed with hot water, sweetened with a spoonful of Manuka active honey. Even if you don't have a cold, this is just beautiful on a cold winter's night.

Manuka Honey is different from other honeys in that it contains an extra, naturally occurring active ingredient known as UMF (Unique Manuka Factor) and the higher the number the better the health benefits it gives. The antiviral and antibacterial actions can be very useful with colds and sore throats.

Ginger is nature's super-root (or rhizome to be VERY pedantic) and seemingly fights almost every common aliment, which is why we have it in the J'M-sip. Ginger is

known to be effective for the treatment of cataracts, amenorrhoea, heart disease, migraines, stroke, angina, athlete's foot, colds, bursitis, chronic fatigue, tendinitis, flu, coughs, depression, dizziness, fever, erectile difficulties, infertility, kidney stones, Raynaud's disease, sciatica, viral infections and the list goes on and on...

Lemon juice is very high in citric acid, which has been documented over the years as helping the body fight off colds. It's also a liver stimulant and can control irritable bowel syndrome and regulate constipation and diarrhoea. It can also help heartburn, bloating, and gas. As lemon juice contains calcium, it's also good for your bones and teeth and its magnesium content will also help with colds and fevers too. All of which is just perfect if you are lying in bed and feel like you've just been run over by a truck.

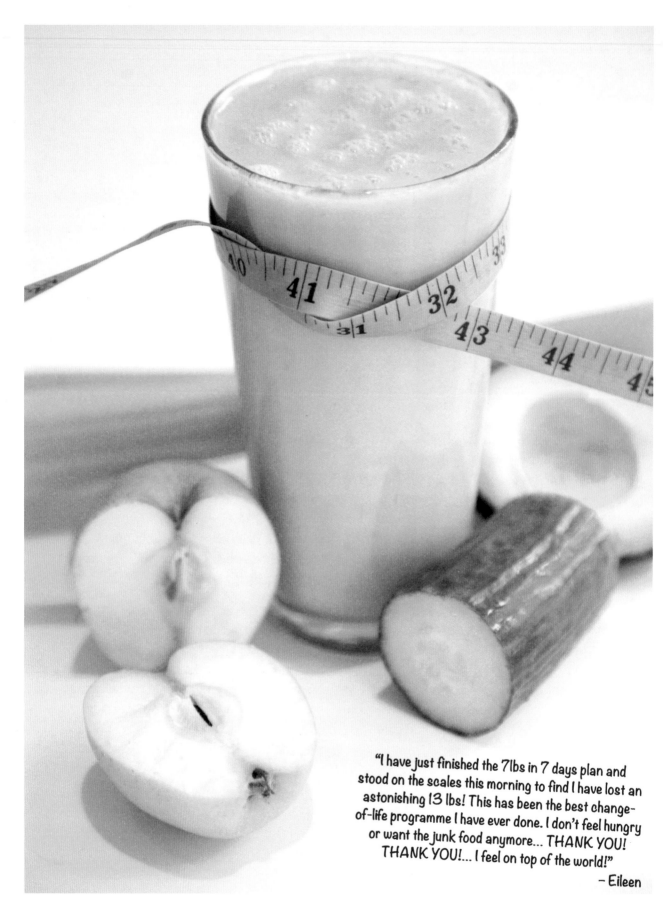

"I have just finished the 7lbs in 7 days plan and stood on the scales this morning to find I have lost an astonishing 13 lbs! This has been the best change-of-life programme I have ever done. I don't feel hungry or want the junk food anymore... THANK YOU! THANK YOU!... I feel on top of the world!"

– Eileen

Slimming Smoothie
The One For Weight Loss

PRESCRIPTION
FOLLOW DIRECTIONS BELOW
TO BE TAKEN AS REQUIRED

JHS
Juicy Health Service

Apples
TWO GOLDEN DELICIOUS

Celery
TWO STALKS

Cucumber
ONE-THIRD MEDIUM

Lime
ONE (PEELED)

Fresh Ginger Root
3 CM CHUNK

Avocado
ONE-HALF (RIPE)

Ice Cubes
SMALL HANDFUL

INSTRUCTIONS: Juice the apples, celery, cucumber, lime, and ginger. Place the juice, ice and avocado into the blender, and blend until smooth.

BEST SERVED: as a meal replacement for breakfast. When you wake up, take on board some hot water and lemon, and go for a run. If you workout on an empty stomach in the morning you turn into a "fat burning machine"! You will be amazed at what a difference a little workout and this smoothie (as a meal replacement) once or twice a day, will have on your waistline and overall health.

Of all the ways to lose weight, I do not know of a more guaranteed or healthier way to do it than a well thought out fresh juicing programme. My *7lbs in 7 Days, Super Juice Diet* book has sold over 1 million copies.

I have received thousands of emails from people all over the world who have not only lost 7-18 lbs in just seven days, but reached their goal weight and moreover, kept it off.

These emails aren't from one or two people, but from thousands all over the world. You will see some examples in the "Community Juice" section. It is also worth catching up with Joe Cross and Phil Staple's stories in the inspirational documentary *Fat, Sick and Nearly Dead*. If you do ever follow my juice "diet", I would advise watching this documentary before you start.

If you don't fancy doing a juicing programme and want just a "meal replacement" smoothie to help you lose weight gradually – here it is! The Slimming Smoothie has been carefully designed to provide your body with the right essential fats, carbohydrates, amino acids, vitamins, minerals, water and enzymes - the right fuel to keep you sustained. If you replace your breakfast with this smoothie, it should keep your hunger at bay 'til at least lunch. If you eat three times a day, you have totally transformed 33% of your daily intake to a no dairy, no wheat, no refined sugar, no trans or saturated fats, no artificial flavour, no artificial sweeteners, 100% pure plant based meal. Replace two meals a day with this and another smoothie from this book, you've hit 66%. Follow that with an evening carb-free meal (perhaps some fish and salad) and you'll be on your way to the land of the slim and trim in no time at all!

"Dear Jason, well I have to be honest from the start – I really didn't think I would be one of the people e-mailing you with such incredible results. I have just completed 7lbs in 7 days and am happy to let you know the results. Here is the amazing part! In 7 days I lost 2¼ inches from chest, 3-4 inches from my hips and 2¾ inches from my waist (I have moved 3 notches on my belt) Then the truly fantastic result – I had lost 18 lbs in 1 week – yes eighteen!!! Thank you Jason"

– Andy W

It's even a best selling app now!

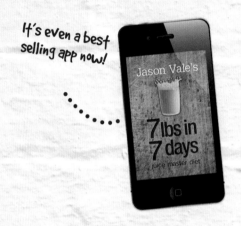

"In seven days I was 9 pounds lighter, my skin softer, mind clearer, energy levels better than they've been in years (I've just hit 40) and my jeans fitted me again. Phew. Jason Vale's message is clear, simple and loaded with common sense. It really does change and hone the way you approach your food and your health. The weight has stayed off, I juice everyday now and the changes in my life has been incredibly positive - and I'm one of life's sceptics. So do yourself a favour, get reading, get juicing and get happy…"

– Q (Amazon review)

"…I woke up on day 8 and after the 7lbs in 7 days plan, weighed myself and found I'd lost 13 lbs. I didn't feel hungry, I was not tired and I did not crave anything during the week. I actually found the 7 days quite easy and enjoyable; day 2-4 I did have a headache but I put that down to caffeine withdrawal. I am now continuing with the Turbo Charge Your Life In 14 Days plan and I have to say I really enjoy having the juices in the morning, but I love all the lunch and dinner recipes too. This one is definitely not a diet, but a 'wake up and look what we've been doing to ourselves and isn't it time we put some thought into our lifestyle' plan…"

– G Cleeve

"…I got on the scales this morning. I had to get off again as I thought the scale was broken. Got back on and my jaw dropped. I lost 15 lbs! …I can't thank you enough…"
– Gary

"I love this programme and I lost almost 11 lbs in 7 days! I was so excited that I carried on doing it for another week and lost 5 lbs more…"
– Sunshine

"I followed this to the letter and I lost 8 lbs in 7 days. I also lost 7 cm around my waist and 6 cm around my hips. I never once felt hungry or felt fatigued and I managed to do between 35 minutes and 60 minutes of exercise every day…"
– Mrs B

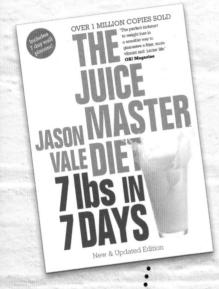

Look it's the updated version of my best-selling 7lbs in 7 Days Super Juice Diet, it's gone all funky and fresh looking and now comes with a free 7 day wall-planner!

It used to look like this…. Now it's gone all funky

This book even knocked The Da Vinci Code off the number one spot. How cool!

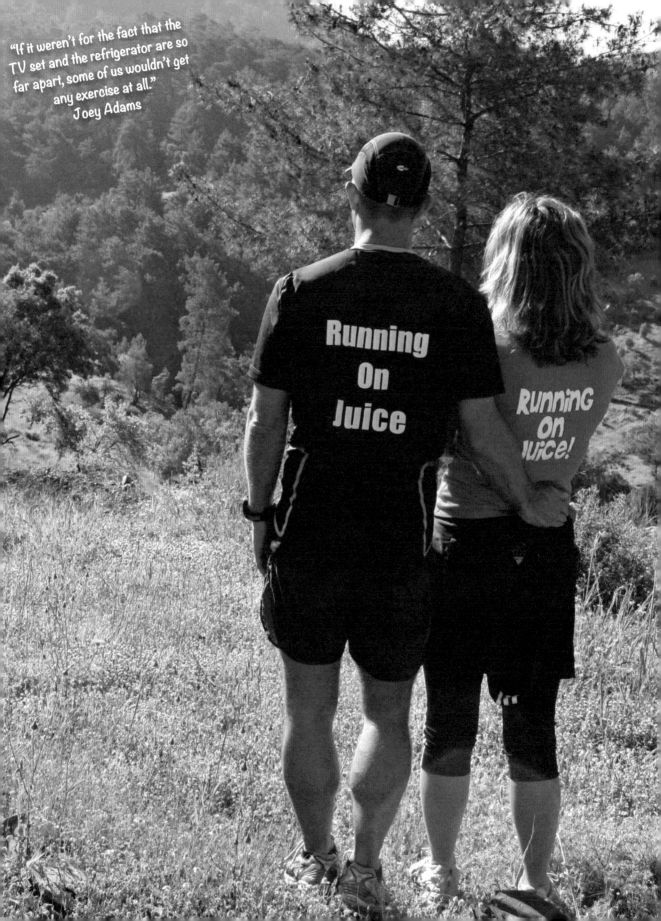

"If it weren't for the fact that the TV set and the refrigerator are so far apart, some of us wouldn't get any exercise at all."
Joey Adams

Gym Bunny
"Possible Is Everything!"

At Juicy HQ we like to move about a bit and keep active. It helps to keep us alert, healthy and out of too much trouble. We tend to go for a nice bounce on our super wonderful mini trampolines. However, whatever exercise you choose, it can produce damaging free radicals plus some aches and pains, especially if you haven't done any for a while.

Liquid Engineering For Your Body

The following juices and smoothies have been carefully designed for you gym bunnies out there. They contain the perfect balance of potassium and sodium (for the muscles), are loaded with nitrates (helps to open the blood vessels and supply more oxygen for working out) and all have plenty of antioxidants, needed for countering any adverse free radical damage.

So get juicing and get bouncing!… or running, or walking, or biking, or lifting weights, or doing aerobics (where you do moves like "grapevine"), or Bikram Yoga (which is really hot)… or…

Okay! I think you've got the picture!

"PAIN IS TEMPORARY QUITTING LASTS A LIFETIME"
LANCE ARMSTRONG

"SO I SAID TO THE GYM INSTRUCTOR: 'CAN YOU TEACH ME TO DO THE SPLITS?' HE SAID: 'HOW FLEXIBLE ARE YOU?' I SAID: 'I CAN'T MAKE TUESDAYS.'"
TIM VINE

"SOME PEOPLE LIKE GOING TO THE PUB; I ENJOY GOING TO THE GYM."
FRANK BRUNO

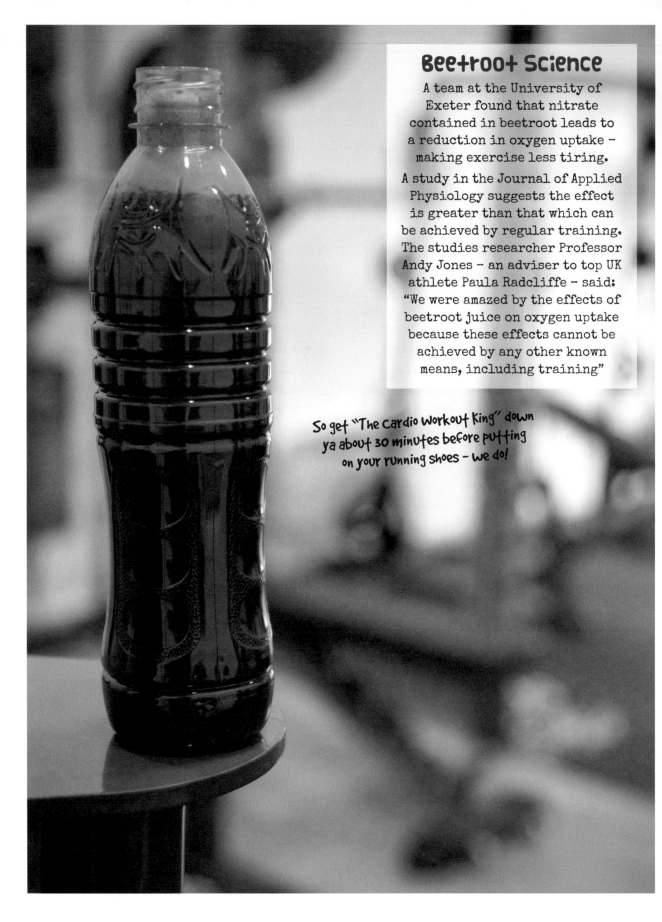

Beetroot Science

A team at the University of Exeter found that nitrate contained in beetroot leads to a reduction in oxygen uptake – making exercise less tiring.

A study in the Journal of Applied Physiology suggests the effect is greater than that which can be achieved by regular training. The studies researcher Professor Andy Jones – an adviser to top UK athlete Paula Radcliffe – said: "We were amazed by the effects of beetroot juice on oxygen uptake because these effects cannot be achieved by any other known means, including training"

So get "The Cardio Workout King" down ya about 30 minutes before putting on your running shoes – we do!

The Cardio Workout King

All hail the king of juices for pre and post cardio workout.

Raw Beetroot
1 medium

Celery
1 stick

Cucumber
¼ medium

Golden Delicious Apple
1

Dr. Martins' Coconut Water
250 ml

Ice Cubes
1 small handful

Work it, Baby!

Juice the beetroot, celery, cucumber and apple.

Add the juice to the blender along with the coconut water and ice. Blend until ready.

Best Served… take half your juice about 30 minutes before a workout and the rest from a flask once you have finished and you are sitting in a nice hot sauna!

Why Dr. Martins coco Juice?

Dr. Antonio Martins' Coco Juice is tapped directly from fresh, organic coconuts using a patented process to ensure the coconut water never comes into contact with light or air. In other words, they've fooled the juice into thinking it's still inside the coconut! So you can have 100% genuine, live, fresh coconut water without having to climb a single palm tree – which is quite neat.

It's also worth knowing that the coconut water is isotonic (will replace the fluids and minerals lost when the body exercises), which is always good when it comes to getting physical.

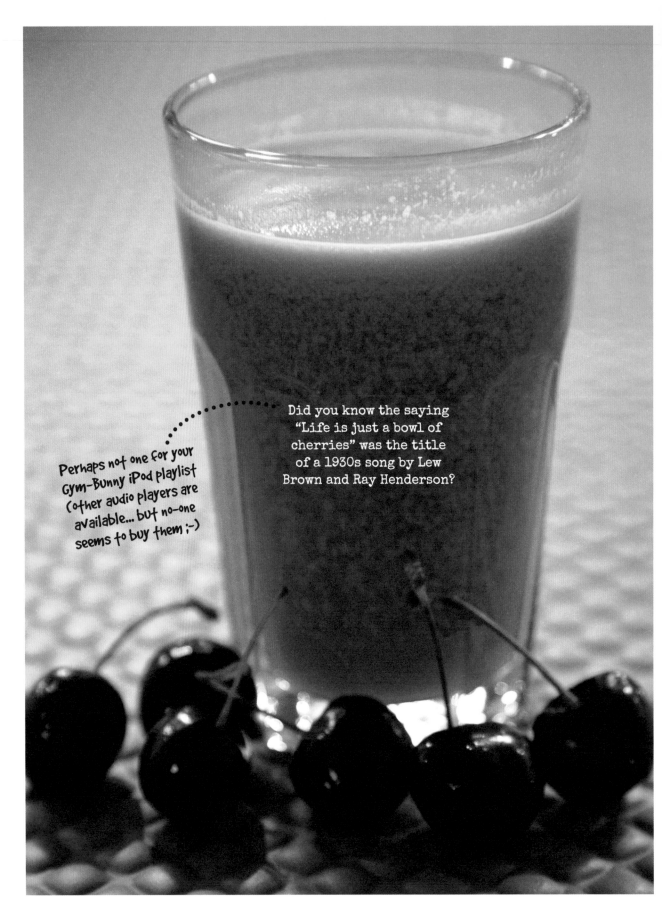

Cherry Toning Tonic

The perfect smoothie for **helping your muscles recover** after that class you took that made you use almost every muscle in your body – including ones you didn't even know you had!

Cherries
15 (pitted)

Dr. Martins' Coconut Water
500 ml

Ice Cubes
1 small handful

Time To Get Toned

Make sure you remove the pits from the cherries – they won't make your juicer very happy.

Add all the ingredients to the blender and blend until smooth.

Best Served... in a sports water bottle directly after your toning workout. Equally as good after some cardio too, it is naturally isotonic, after all!

Life Is A Bowl of Cherries

A study conducted at London's South Bank University found that consuming cherry juice improved the recovery of muscle strength after intense exercise. In the study the maximum voluntary muscle contraction of subjects who consumed cherry juice for one week before and two days after a series of single leg knee extensions recovered significantly faster than those who didn't.

So okay, the cherries do need pitting, but it's so worth it!

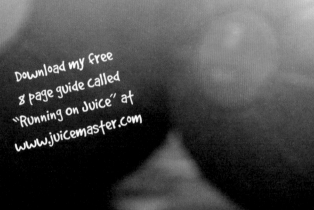

Download my free
8 page guide called
"Running On Juice" at
www.juicemaster.com

Why IS The Marathon 26.2 Miles?

Because that's roughly the distance between the Greek cities of Marathon and Athens. In 490 B.C. the Greek army repelled a Persian naval invasion on the plains surrounding the coastal city of Marathon. According to legend, a runner was sent to Athens to relay news of the victory. Upon reaching Athens, the young man shouted "Rejoice, we conquer!" and fell to the ground dead. So the first person to ever run a marathon died – no wonder I found it tough!

Not strictly true, he actually fell to his death after he ran there and back!

Juice Master's Marathon Smoothie

This smoothie is perfect before a full or half marathon. I have run the London and New York marathons and the Great North Run every year. One to two hours before each race, I tuck into one of these as it contains amino acids, carbohydrates, essential fats, vitamins, minerals, enzymes and water. It has an ideal balance of sodium and potassium and **perfect for long-distance running**.

Pineapple
2 cm slice

Golden Delicious Apples
3

Celery
2 sticks

Raw Beetroot
1 bulb

Lime
1 (peeled)

Cucumber
⅓ medium

Avocado
1 small (ripe)

Banana
1 (ripe & peeled)

Juice Master's Hemp Protein Power
1 teaspoon (optional)

Ice Cubes
1 small handful

Ready... Set... Go!

Peel the lime, leaving as much of the nutrient-rich white pith as possible.

Juice the pineapple (no need to peel if you have a good juicer), apples, celery, beetroot, lime, and cucumber.

Put the avocado into the blender along with the peeled banana, protein powder and the ice. Blend until smooth. If it's too thick, simply add more apple juice.

Best Served... in a flask and drink 1–2 hours before a long race.

You Can't Beet This Science!

Researchers from Exeter University and Peninsula Medical School in Devon found that raw beetroot juice contains high levels of nitrate, which widens the blood vessels, reducing blood pressure and allowing more blood flow. It actually cuts the amount of oxygen needed by your muscles, even during low-intensity exercise.

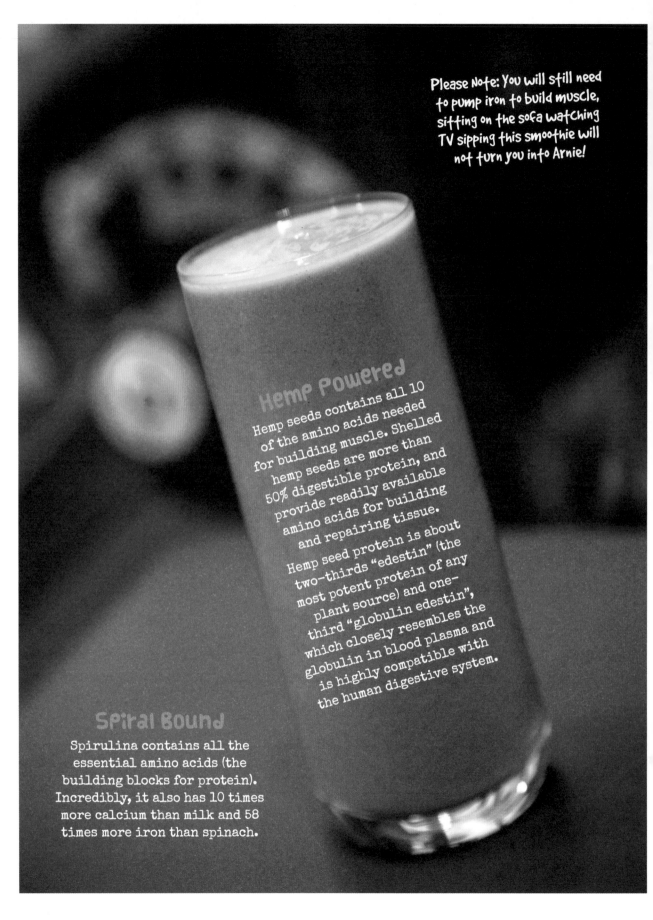

Please Note: You will still need to pump iron to build muscle, sitting on the sofa watching TV sipping this smoothie will not turn you into Arnie!

Hemp Powered

Hemp seeds contains all 10 of the amino acids needed for building muscle. Shelled hemp seeds are more than 50% digestible protein, and provide readily available amino acids for building and repairing tissue. Hemp seed protein is about two-thirds "edestin" (the most potent protein of any plant source) and one-third "globulin edestin", which closely resembles the globulin in blood plasma and is highly compatible with the human digestive system.

Spiral Bound

Spirulina contains all the essential amino acids (the building blocks for protein). Incredibly, it also has 10 times more calcium than milk and 58 times more iron than spinach.

Pure Muscle Builder

Did you know, the largest land animals on Earth with the biggest muscles are all vegan. So you don't necessarily need animal protein to build human muscle. Your body also builds muscle from amino acids – found in all plant foods

This "Pure Muscle Builder" smoothie contains **every single essential amino acid** the body needs.

Golden Delicious Apples
2

Spinach Leaves
1 large handful

Pineapple
⅓ medium

Avocado
1 medium (ripe)

Spirulina
1 teaspoon

Juice Master's Hemp Protein Power
1 heaped teaspoon (optional)

Ice Cubes
1 small handful

Start Building Those Muscles

Juice the apples, spinach and pineapple (no need to peel if you have a good juicer). Before you turn the juicer on, make sure you pack the spinach tightly into the chute, behind the apple, to get maximum juice.

Pour the fresh juice into the blender then add the avocado, spirulina, hemp powder and ice. Blend until smooth making sure all the powder has been fully dissolved.

Best Served... in your favourite flask, about one hour after lifting weights in order to feed those torn muscles.

Bursting with nutrients

Avocados are packed with practically everything your body needs. They contain vitamins A, B-complex, C, E, H, K, and folic acid; plus magnesium, copper, iron, calcium, potassium and many other trace elements. Avocados also provide all of the essential amino acids, plus 7 fatty acids, including omega 3 and 6, and more protein than cows' milk. All that and they make your smoothies creamier!

"The last three or four reps is what makes the muscle grow. This area of pain divides the champion from someone else who is not a champion. That's what most people lack, having the guts to go on and just say they'll go through the pain no matter what happens."
Arnold Schwarzenegger

Summer breeze makes me feel fine
Blowin' through the jasmine in my mind
Summer juice makes me feel fine
Feeding every cell in my body and mind
(Isley Brothers... with a little
input from Juice Master Jay!)

We LOVE summer,
made even lovelier with
some fresh juice!

COOL SUMMER JUICES

When summer is in the air there's no better way to cool down than with a beautiful, freshly extracted, healthy juice. Together with the Juice Master team, I have created ten of the finest summer coolers for your pleasure. No blender or supplements required – just juice the ingredients and pour over ice.

FRESH MINT LEMONADE

OLYMPIC STRENGTH

ANYONE FOR TENNIS

GET RIPPED

SUMMERTIME BLUES

SUMMER SLIMMER

SUMMER LOVIN'

THE HEALTHY MOJITO

LOLLY IN A GLASS

BITTER-SWEET SUNSHINE

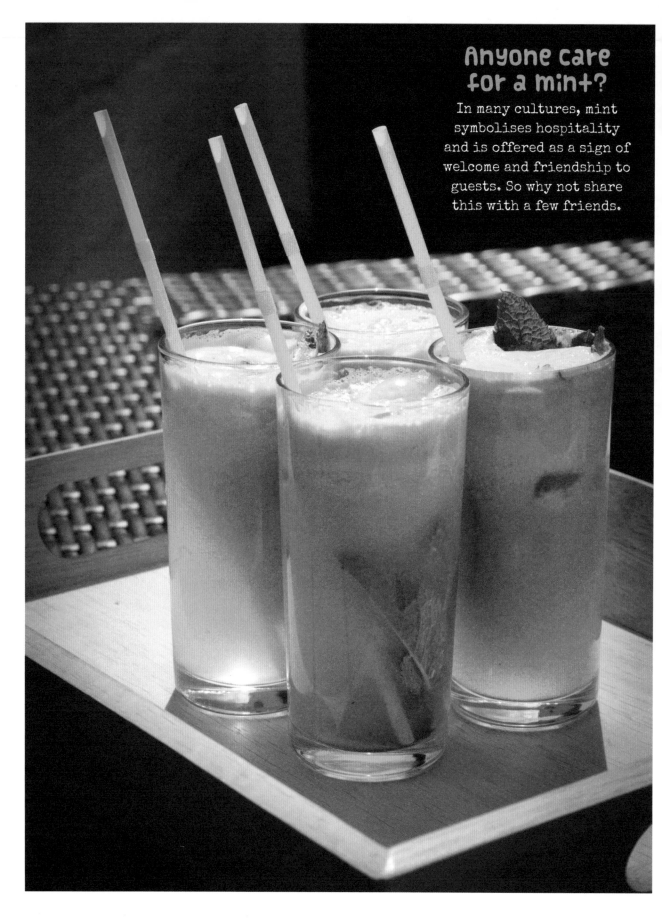

Anyone care for a mint?

In many cultures, mint symbolises hospitality and is offered as a sign of welcome and friendship to guests. So why not share this with a few friends.

Fresh Mint Lemonade

It's the world famous Juice Master Lemon...Aid but with a **delicious minty twist**. You will not believe how deliciously fresh this juice tastes!

Golden Delicious Apple
2

Lemon
⅓ medium

Fresh Mint Leaves
1 handful

Ice Cubes
1 small handful

Get the juice party started this summer!

Put one apple into the chute, pack in the mint and lemon and then finish with the other apple. Juice the lot and pour over ice and mint.

Best Served... If you are having a BBQ this summer why not do something a little different. Simply set up your juicer to the side of the BBQ or at the 'kitchen hub' (where most people end up) along with a load of apples, lemons, fresh mint, glasses and ice and get your guests to make their own 'homemade mint lemonade' It's a wonderful talking point, it's interactive, it's fun and it helps to get the party going. Plus the little ones will LOVE it, as it tastes just like lemonade but without the refined sugar.

Not Just A Cool Taste

Peppermint is one of the oldest (and best tasting) natural remedies for indigestion. Studies have found that peppermint stimulates the gastric lining to produce enzymes which aid digestion and lessen the amount of time food spends in the stomach.

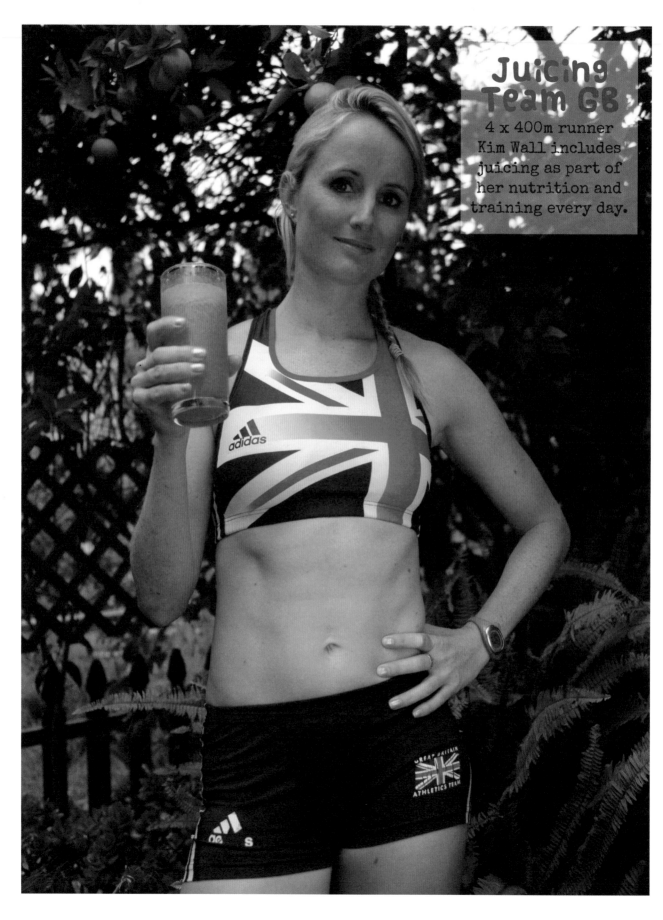

Juicing
Team GB

4 x 400m runner
Kim Wall includes
juicing as part of
her nutrition and
training every day.

Olympic Strength

Congratulations to team GB at the 2012 London Olympic games – you made us all very proud! If the games inspired you to peak performance, then do as some of the athletes did when training, juice up! Here's a **nutrient rich powerhouse** of a juice to help you run like a (Usain) Bolt!

Golden Delicious Apples
2

Raw Beetroot
1/2 bulb

Spinach
1 large handful

Lemon
1/3 (peeled)

Ice Cubes
1 small handful

Build Natural Strength

Pack the chute with one of the apples, then follow with the beetroot, spinach (make sure it's washed) and lemon. Top off the chute with the final apple, turn the machine on push the lot through!

Best Served... running through the streets of London, carrying the Olympic torch, while crowds of people cheer and wave as you triumphantly enter Wembley Stadium.

Juicing for Great Britain!

Juice Master had been asked to work with some of the Olympic runners and hockey players to incorporate juices into their training for the London 2012 Olympics.

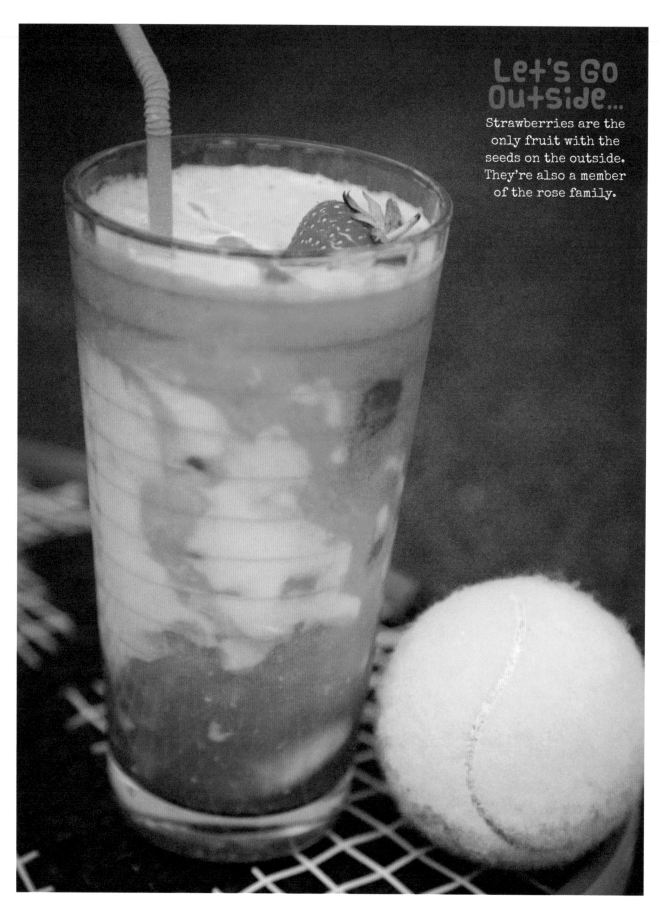

Let's Go Outside...

Strawberries are the only fruit with the seeds on the outside. They're also a member of the rose family.

Anyone for Tennis?

When Wimbledon is in full flow, there's nothing tastier and more British than a good serving of strawberries and cream. No cream in this juice though, we've replaced it with low fat yogurt. I think you're going to be pleasantly surprised, in fact you're going to **"forty-love"** it!

Fresh Strawberries
400g

Pineapple
½ (peeled)

Live Yogurt or Soya Yogurt
4 tablespoons

Ice Cubes
1 small handful

"Serve" yourself this tennis treat

Pack the strawberries into the chute before you turn on the machine. Juice on the slowest setting and push through slowly so you extract as much juice possible. Juice the pineapple on the fastest speed setting. Half fill a tall glass with juice, add two tablespoons of yogurt, top up with juice then add the rest of the yogurt. Swirl round with a spoon and enjoy.

Best Served... Whilst sitting in the sun on an English lawn watching Wimbledon on you tablet (FYI summer in the UK usually falls on a Thursday afternoon in mid-July!).

That's a Lotta Fruit!

Hugh Lowe Farms in Kent, provides 30 tonnes of strawberries to Wimbledon over the fortnight. They've been the only provider of Wimbledon strawberries for over 20 years.

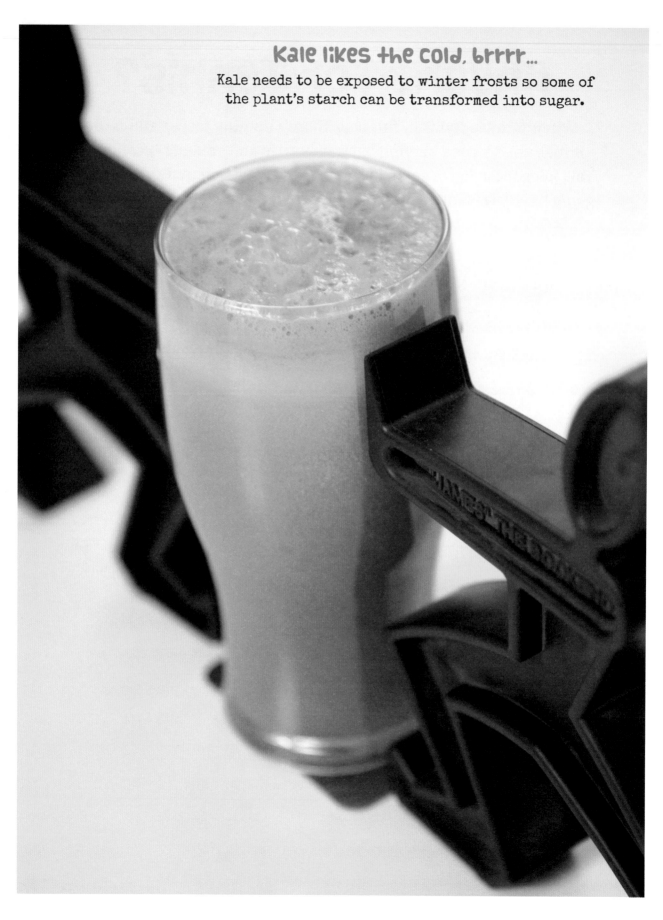

Kale likes the cold, brrrr...

Kale needs to be exposed to winter frosts so some of
the plant's starch can be transformed into sugar.

Get Ripped

It's summertime and the summer holidays signal a time of beaches, ice creams, sand, sea and surf. Tone up and achieve that ripped body you've always wanted with this **super green, super healthy** juice.

Golden Delicious Apples
2

Celery
1 stick

Cucumber
¼ medium

Spinach
1 small handful

Kale
1 small handful

Ice Cubes
1 small handful

Get ready to get ripped

Put the apple in first. Pack all of the other ingredients into the chute and then use the second apple to pack everything in tight.

Juice everything on the highest setting on your juicer and pour over ice.

Best Served... If you, like many, are doing that little bit of exercise to look your best for the beach, then drink this juice, just before and after training to help you feed your muscles.

Vitamin K-ale!

Kale is high in vitamin K, vitamin C and carotenoids. It also contains sulforaphane which has been studied for it's anti-cancer properties; and indole-3-carbinol which boosts DNA repair in cells.

A Popular Berry

Blueberries are a very popular
fruit. Last year over 1,500
new products were introduced
containing blueberries.

Summertime Blues

To say I am a fan of Eddie Cochran is perhaps an understatement. One of his classic tracks has the lyrics "there ain't no cure for the summertime blues". Well I beg to differ on that one Eddie as this juice not only *tastes amazing* but has also been designed to *cure those summertimes blues!*

Blueberries
2 large handfuls

Blackberries
1 large handful

Oranges
2 (peeled)

Ice Cubes
1 small handful

Juice up this Blues Blaster

Peel the oranges leaving on as much white pith as possible. Place one orange in the juicer chute before turning it on, pack in the berries and finish with the other orange. Juice on the slowest setting. Pour over ice and enjoy.

Best Served... Relax, leave your troubles behind and lift your mood with some juiced food!

Naturally High in Antioxidants

A study conducted by the National Institute of Health found that the anthocyanins in berries inhibit key enzymes that lead to anxiety and depression.

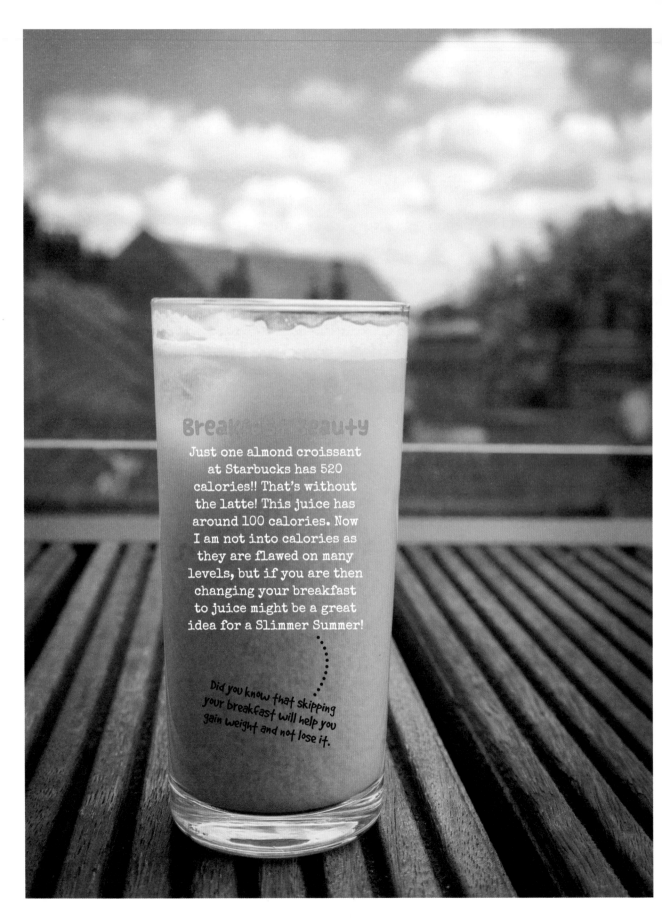

Breakfast Beauty

Just one almond croissant at Starbucks has 520 calories!! That's without the latte! This juice has around 100 calories. Now I am not into calories as they are flawed on many levels, but if you are then changing your breakfast to juice might be a great idea for a Slimmer Summer!

Did you know that skipping your breakfast will help you gain weight and not lose it.

Summer Slimmer

When summer first hits it can be good and bad news. On one side, **"YEAH! *The sun's out*"** but on the other, "shoot it's time to wear less and *reveal a bit more!*" Simply change your breakfast to the Summer Slimmer for one week and there should be less of you as a result :)

Pink Lady Apple
2

Cucumber
¼ medium

Celery
1 stick

Raw Ginger Root
3 cm piece

Ice Cubes
1 small handful

The Juicy Way To A Slimmer You!

Put an apples into the chute, followed by the other ingredients and then the other apple. Juice the lot! Pour over ice.

Best Served...

on a hot summers day, a slight breeze blowing over your skin, relaxing in your favourite recliner, on your balcony overlooking the park, listening to the gentle murmur of the world passing you by as you relax and sip this cool, green, super, Summer, Slimmer.

Super Slimming Foods

Did you know that celery has 5 calorie intake, but it takes 10 calories to digest it! And cucumber is a natural diuretic, it helps to 'flush' excess toxicity from the body – both of which aids weight loss.

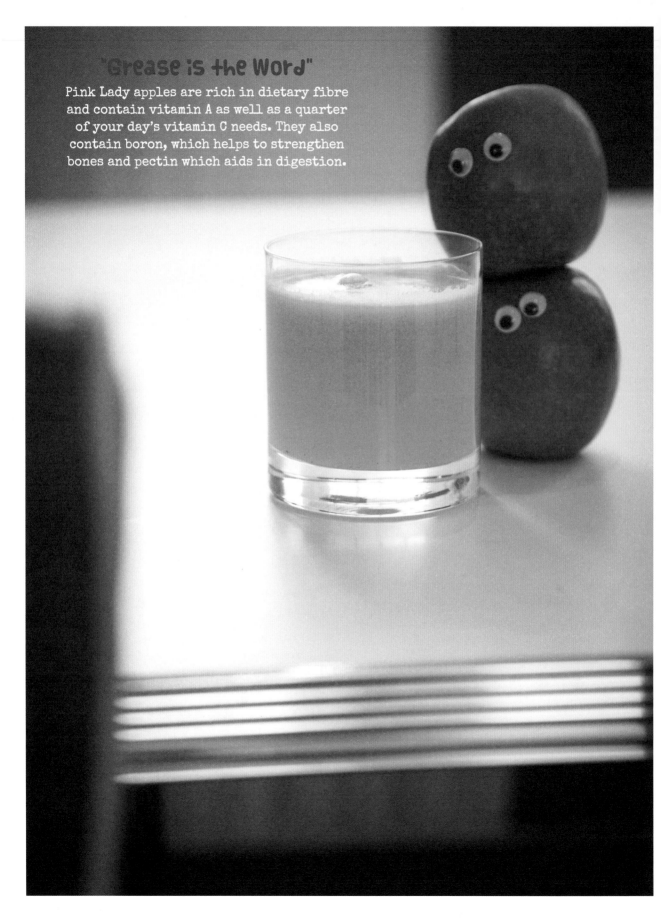

"Grease is the Word"

Pink Lady apples are rich in dietary fibre and contain vitamin A as well as a quarter of your day's vitamin C needs. They also contain boron, which helps to strengthen bones and pectin which aids in digestion.

Summer Lovin'

Take yourself back to the **_"Summer of Fun"_**, with the T-Birds and Pink Ladies having **_"A Blast"_**. I even had a black leather T-Bird jacket when I was eight years old and could be seen dancing round Peckham like a young Danny Zuko!

Pink Lady Apple
1

Pear
1 medium

Parsnip
1 small

Fresh Mint Leaves
1 handful

Ice Cubes
1 small handful

"You better shape up"

Load the pear and parsnip in the chute, then pack in the mint behind it. Place the apple behind the mint and juice the lot, pour over ice and enjoy.

Best Served... In an open top Cadillac at a drive-in movie, taking sips in between singing "Grease Lightning" at the top of your voice. Also recommended if you happen to be "stranded at the drive-in and branded a fool!".

Under My Umbelliferae...

The Umbelliferae family, named for its umbrella-like flower clusters, includes celery, carrots and parsnips.

Cool Parsnips!

The unique spicy-sweet flavour comes from the first frost which converts its starches to sugar.

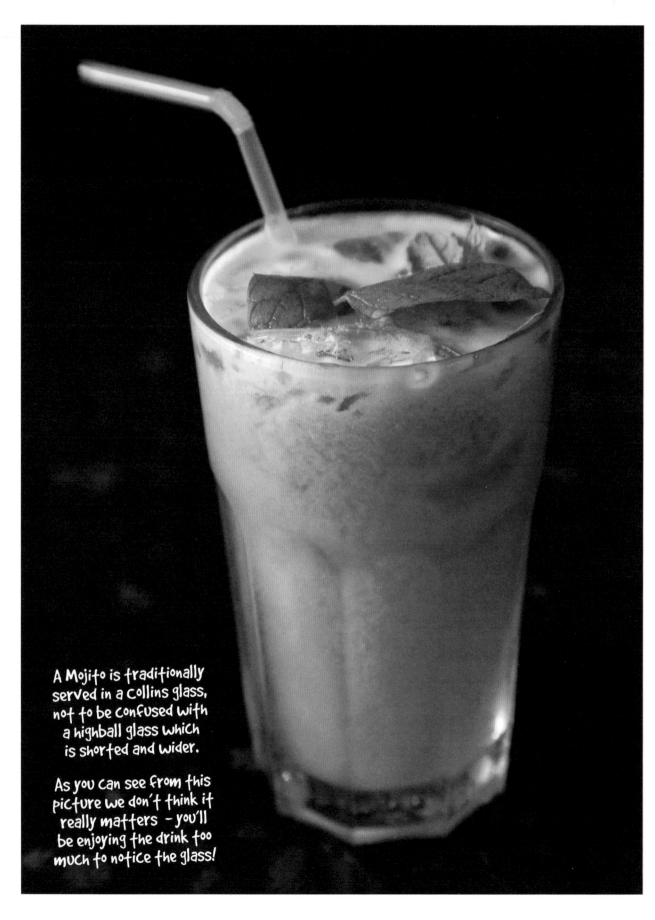

A Mojito is traditionally served in a Collins glass, not to be confused with a highball glass which is shorted and wider.

As you can see from this picture we don't think it really matters - you'll be enjoying the drink too much to notice the glass!

The Healthy Mojito

The Mojito is a cocktail that consists of five ingredients: white rum, sugar, lime juice, sparkling water and mint. In this juice inspired virgin alternative, you can **sip this summertime classic** knowing there's nothing but pure health in your glass.

Lime
1 (peeled)

Fresh Mint Leaves
2 handfuls

Green Seedless Grapes
4 handfuls

Crushed Ice Cubes
1 small handful

A Summertime favourite - made the healthy way!

Line the inside of a tall glass with a handful of mint leaves and fill with crushed ice.

Put the grapes into your juicer with the lime and a handful of mint. Turn your juicer onto the slowest speed setting and push through slowly.

Pour slowly into your glass, garnish with a lime wedge and some mint leaves and serve with a straw. Perfection!

Best Served... In a proper Mojito glass, preferably under a shady palm tree on the gorgeous white sands of Cuba's Playa Paraíso, reading something by Ernest Hemmingway for that little sophisticated touch!

What's in a Name?

There are 2 main theories about the name "Mojito".... One claims it comes from the word "Mojo", which is a Cuban seasoning made from lime juice used to flavour dishes. The other theory is that it comes from the Spanish word "mojado", which means wet.

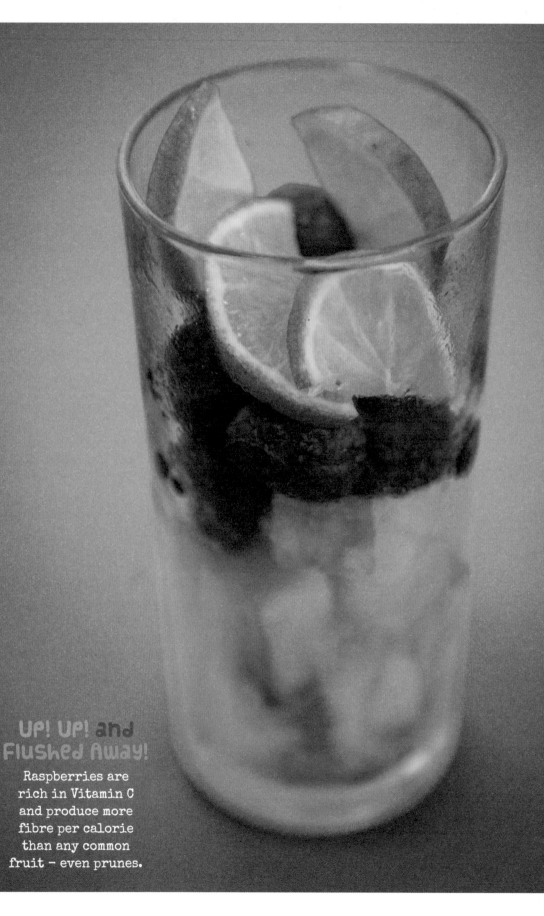

UP! UP! and Flushed Away!

Raspberries are rich in Vitamin C and produce more fibre per calorie than any common fruit – even prunes.

Lolly in a Glass

The chime of the ice cream van is bound to stir your taste buds for a Mr Whippy or a sugary lolly loaded with artificial chemicals and sugars. Why not opt to make your own lolly flavoured juice instead? Or why not freeze the juice in a lolly holder and **enjoy on a hot summers day!**

Lime
⅓ (peeled)

Fresh Raspberries
400g

Pineapple
1/3 (peeled)

Ice Cubes
1 small handful

Lip smackingly delicious with a zesty zing

Pack the raspberries into the chute, then turn the juicer to the slow speed and push through slowly. Crank up your juicer to the highest speed and blitz through the lime and pineapple.

Pour over ice and enjoy as a juice or freeze into lollies, the perfect treat for young and old a like.

Best Served... listening to Greensleeves to bring back those nostalgic memories of running for the ice cream van, a few coins in your hand, crazy with anticipation for a tasty cold treat on a hot summers day. Except this time you don't have to worry that what you're eating isn't good for you.

Did you know...

There are over 200 species of raspberries. Raspberries are available in four different colours. Although red and black are the most common, they can also be purple or even yellow.

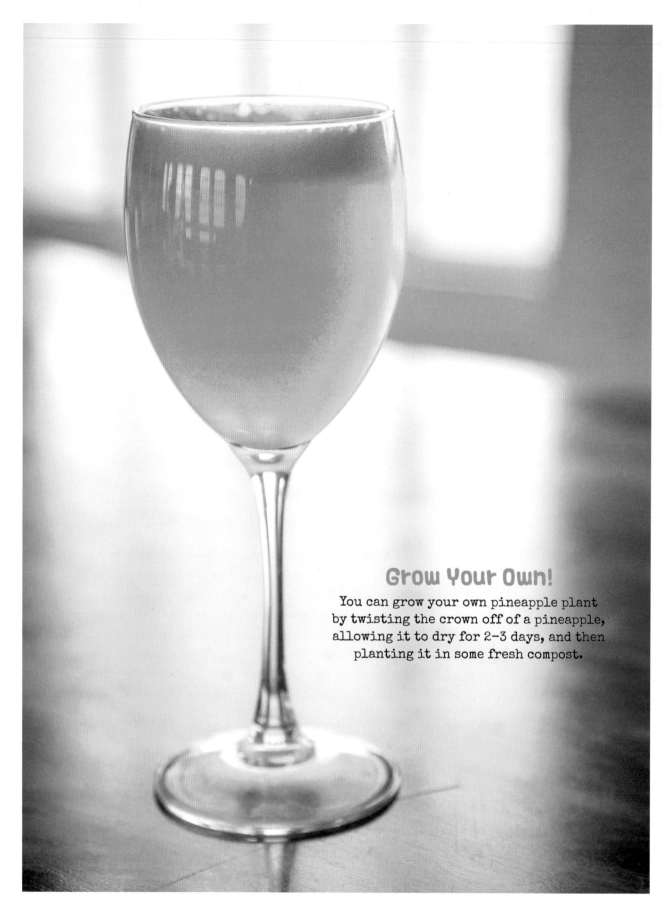

Grow Your Own!

You can grow your own pineapple plant
by twisting the crown off of a pineapple,
allowing it to dry for 2–3 days, and then
planting it in some fresh compost.

Bitter-Sweet Sunshine

There is a drink which resembles this juice but comes in a can and is loaded with refined sugar! You know... the one with **"the totally tropical taste"**.

This refreshing beauty on the other hand, is **as pure as nature herself**.

Pink Grapefruit
½ (peeled)

Pineapple
⅓ (peeled)

San Pellegrino Sparkling Water
300ml

Ice Cubes
1 small handful

Taste Pure Sunshine

Simply juice the grapefruit and pineapple and mix half and half with the sparkling water. Pour over ice and drink.

Best Served... whilst sun bathing on the white sands of a Caribbean paradise, the crystal clear waves lapping against the shore... pure bliss.

Powerful Pineapple

Pineapples contain protein digesting enzymes. The main one is called Bromelain – this stuff is so powerful it is capable of digesting 1000 times its weight of protein. The enzyme also helps to dissolve excess mucus and thus helps to relieve the symptoms of asthma and hay fever.

It takes 18 months or more for a pineapple plant to produce it's first fruit, and each plant only produces one or two pineapples a year.

Known Celebrity Juicers:

JENNIFER ANISTON

ELLEN PAGE

NICOLE RICHIE

PEACHES GELDOLF

GWYNETH PALTROW

WHITNEY PORT

KYLIE MINOGUE

TRACY ANDERSON

BONO

SEAN CONNERY

SIR ANTHONY HOPKINS

OLIVIA WILDE

KATIE PRICE

SARAH JESSICA PARKER

CAPRICE

SIMON COWELL

JESSICA SZOHR

And Many More...

Celebrity Juice!

It seems anyone who is anyone has got the juicing bug. In this section I have included some amazing recipes from some of my "celeb" friends. They have kindly taken time out of their busy lives to come up with a scrummy recipe for the world to share. I have also added a couple of recipes from celebs I have never met, like Simon Cowell and the idol that is Mr David Beckham.

Simon Cowell Super Smoothie

I have added the "Super Smoothie" Simon Cowell drinks as it's been scientifically put together by French Scientists (no less), so I thought it was worth putting in.

I have also added a David Beckham Smoothie (one I've completely made up, didn't come from him at all in case you are wondering) as I simply couldn't miss the opportunity to have a recipe where I could use the title:

Blend It Like Beckham

(Oh come on – genius!)

David, if you are reading this and you do make the odd smoothie or have the odd wheatgrass shot, like your good lady wife, send one in as I'd like to include a genuine, David Beckham recipe in the next print-run.

Any road up, have a little flick through this section, read a little about the celeb and share in their favourite juice.

You may be wondering where the guys from the TV show celeb Juice are, like Holly, Fearne, Rufus and Keith Lemon?
Well I did ask but the only reply I got back was from Keith Lemon (Leigh Frances), he wrote - and I quote:

"I don't have a favourite smoothie recipe, my favourite dinosaur though is a diplodocus! That's not any help though is it really?"

Nope not really Keith. Now when are you guys going to get Juice Master onto Celebrity Juice? #justsaying :-)

Katie Price's
Pretty Pink Passion

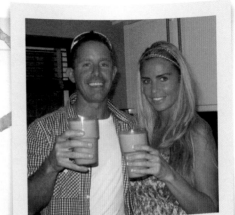

½ medium pineapple
2 apples
2 passion fruit
1 handful strawberries
3 Tbsp bio-live yogurt
ice

Juice the pineapple and apples.
Cut the passion fruits in half and
scoop the flesh into your blender.
Remove the leaves and stalks from
the strawberries and add to the blender along with the yogurt and
ice. Blend until passionately pink and deliciously smooth.

As you can s
– we share t
same passic

Katie Price has become the *Marmite* of the celebrity world – you either love her or don't love her as much – let's just say that! I personally fall into the "love her" camp. Most people only see the "in the press" version of Katie, but the Katie I know is an amazing mother, an extremely hard worker, and someone who has done a great deal to get other people juicing.

I would like to thank Katie for her contribution to my mission to juice the world!

I first met Katie after the birth of her son Junior. With the help of my juicing plan (and her dedication) she lost around 10 kg (22 lbs) in 3 months. News hit several magazines, and as a result many people picked up my *7lbs in 7 Days Super Juice Diet* (also known as *The Juice Master Diet*) and ended

up changing their lives too.

Katie's recipe would be best enjoyed sitting, relaxing while reading one of Katie's 42 books. Yes, at time of writing this page Katie is promoting her 42nd book! I thought I was going some (this book is my 10th) – well done Katie!

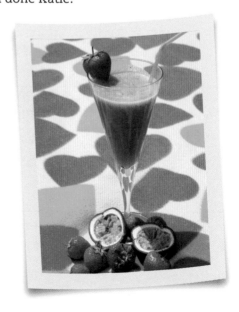

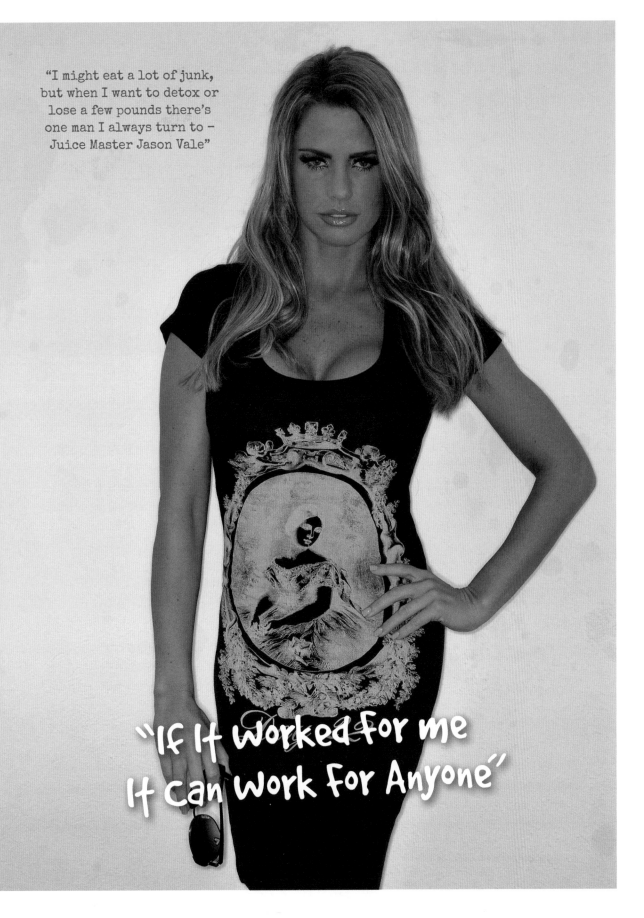

"I might eat a lot of junk, but when I want to detox or lose a few pounds there's one man I always turn to – Juice Master Jason Vale"

"If It Worked For me It can Work For Anyone"

Dedicated to David
Blend It Like Beckham

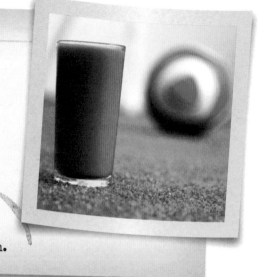

1 medium pineapple   1 raw beetroot
6 sprigs of mint   1 banana
1 tsp Manuka honey
3 tsp bio-live yogurt
ice

Peel the pineapple for this recipe.
Juice the pineapple, beetroot
and mint. Chuck the ice, yogurt,
banana and honey into a blender.
Pour in the juice and blend until smooth.

Don't you just love David Beckham? He is one of life's super nice and very genuine guys. He does so much for so many people, usually behind the scenes. He has been out to see our troops on several occasions, often not telling a soul and just turning up and hanging with them. Not to be the big "I am" but because he is one of life's very rare, genuine people. He is, I feel, one of the finest role models of our time, if not the finest.

Possibly, the Greatest Man To Ever Don The England Shirt

Okay, so he shouldn't be in charge of naming children, but hey, you can't be all things to all people. After all, naming your baby girl Harper Seven (which, if you say it quick enough, sounds like "half past seven") isn't exactly setting the kid up for a life without some challenges in the playground (only kidding David… ish).

Now I have no idea if a juice or smoothie ever passes David's lips, but I understand Victoria has found the juicy light in-so-much as she has been reported as being a bit partial to the odd shot of wheatgrass.

A Juicy Alternative To Oranges At Half Time

However, I have left wheatgrass from this smoothie (most will be pleased to hear) and instead I've created one I feel not only tastes incredible, but is perfect for playing sports, like football for example (or soccer as they call it in the USA. They do this because they already use the word football for another game they play… with their hands! "Go figure!" as they say).

David and Victoria, Posh and Becks, I salute you!

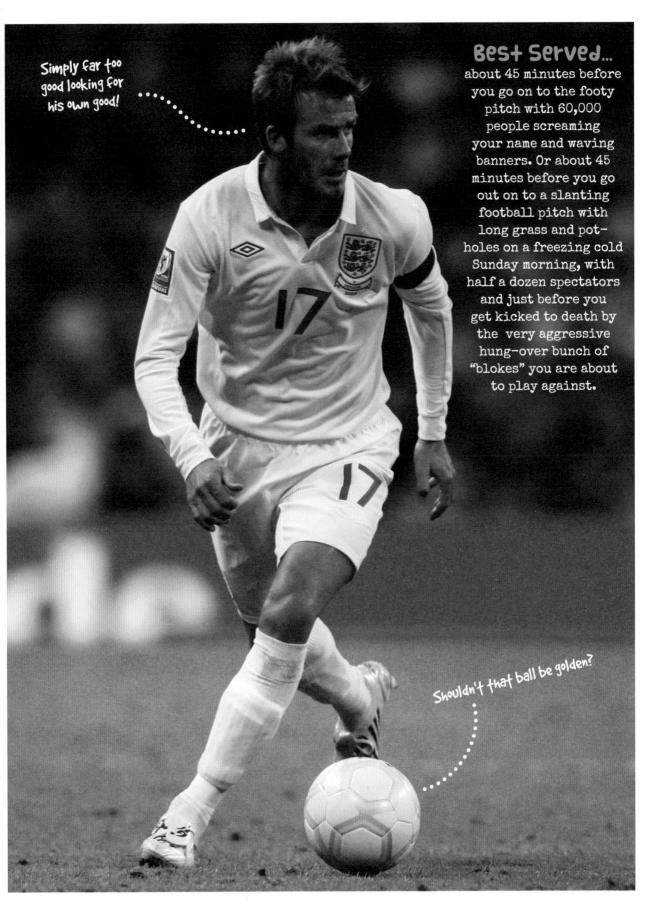

Simply far too good looking for his own good!

Best Served...

about 45 minutes before you go on to the footy pitch with 60,000 people screaming your name and waving banners. Or about 45 minutes before you go out on to a slanting football pitch with long grass and pot-holes on a freezing cold Sunday morning, with half a dozen spectators and just before you get kicked to death by the very aggressive hung-over bunch of "blokes" you are about to play against.

Shouldn't that ball be golden?

Beverley Knight's
Juice With Soul

1 medium raw beetroot
2 golden delicious apples
1 handful spinach leaves
1 handful blackberries (fresh or frozen)
1 handful crushed ice

Juice the beetroot, apples and spinach leaves (remember to pack the leaves in tight between the apples).

Add the juice to the blender along with the blackberries and a handful of ice. Blend until smooth.

I had the amazing good fortune of meeting Beverley Knight at my retreat. I am also sure the rest of the guests that week couldn't believe their luck, especially when Bev got up on the final night and started to sing acapella. It is hard to convey just how good Beverley Knight is with just her and her voice, but everyone had goosebumps.

> "...Juice every day resulted in my skin clearing-up, my eyes and hair shining and dropping 3 kg..."

In my opinion Beverley is right up there with Aretha Franklin and is one of the true greats. There are those who can sing and those who own it; Beverley owns it! At the time of writing Beverley has just released a new album, *SOUL UK*. There are far too many great tracks on it to mention, but her version of George Michael's "One More Try" is, I feel, Beverley at her best. From previous albums I would have to choose her track *GOLD*, which she sang at the retreat and I will never forget it. Actually I could mention loads of her other tracks, like her version of *Piece Of My Heart* – genius. I think the easiest route is to get some of Beverley into your life by jumping online – now – and downloading a few of her albums!

Beverley's New Album Cover Looks Like This

Beverley has kindly added her favourite smoothie for all of us to share. She is a big juicing fan and it's one of the ways she stays looking the way she does – sensational. I have to be careful here as if I'm too complimentary about her figure, her very fit cage fighting fiancé, James, might have a word or two!

"Beetroot is apparently the thing that helps oxygenize the blood, what every performer needs! My juice has lots of iron for strength, hence the spinach. Blackberries? I just love them! Good for the skin, small and sweet like me!"

"The week I spent at the Juice Master retreat was life-changing!"

Lord Phil Harris
Super Juice

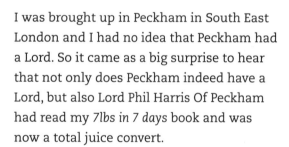

2 golden delicious apples
½ lime (peeled)   ¼ pineapple
¼ medium cucumber   ¼ avocado
1 fl oz shot fresh wheatgrass (or
    1 tsp wheatgrass powder)
1 tsp spirulina
1 capsule acidophilus bacteria powder
ice

Juice the apples, lime, pineapple and cucumber. Pour the juice into a blender with the avocado, wheatgrass and other supplements and don't forget the ice. Blend and enjoy.

I was brought up in Peckham in South East London and I had no idea that Peckham had a Lord. So it came as a big surprise to hear that not only does Peckham indeed have a Lord, but also Lord Phil Harris Of Peckham had read my *7lbs in 7 days* book and was now a total juice convert.

"Unlike other diets I have been on, I never felt hungry or tired..."

Lord Harris hopes his story will inspire others to a juicy way of life. He lost an incredible 42 lbs in just 11 weeks after reading the book. It turns out we have quite a bit in common. We both worked down the market in Peckham and remember when Peckham High Street and Rye Lane were thriving.

In 2007 Lord Harris returned to Peckham and opened a Carpetright (yes he's the chap who owns Carpetright, with 600 stores and counting – not bad for a chap who worked down the market).

"It's a great tool. If I ever put on weight I know I can just juice for a few days and it will drop off..."

Lord Harris does an enormous amount to help Schools in South East London and as I write this, 28 flats above his store in Tottenham, and his store, were completely destroyed in the mindless rioting. Instead of getting angry, he is simply deeply concerned about the people who have lost everything and will be helping them all. That is the kind of true gentleman he is. I am pleased he has found juicing and has dropped the weight and his health is improving dramatically as we need people like Lord Harris to remain in this world for as long as possible.

GOOD LoRD... literally!
Did you know Lord Harris gives millions of pounds to help deprived communities like my old hunting ground Peckham? Well he does, and we thank him for it :-)

(19 kg / 42 lbs)
"I Lost 3 stone in 11 weeks and knocked 3 points off my cholesterol"

Simon Cowell
Super Smoothie

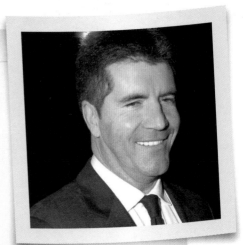

30 red or black grapes
½ golden delicious apple
15 blueberries   9 strawberries
8 lingonberries   5 acerola berries
5 chokeberries

Place the apple into the chute, then add
the grapes and lingonberries, packing
them in tight so you will get more juice.

Pour the juice into the blender. Add all of
the other berries and ice. Blend until smooth.

I haven't personally met Simon, although one day hope to, but I have read a great deal about his anti-aging secrets, one of which being his "Super Smoothie". Well I say his, it was actually created by French scientists, at the University of Strasbourg. They claim this unique combination of seven fruit juices boosts health and cuts the risk of heart disease and stroke.

Simon Cowell's Super Smoothie Was Created By French Scientists

Here you'll find two recipes. One is the actual Simon Cowell smoothie and the other is my version (in the glass on the other page).

In Simon's Smoothie you will find cowberry (otherwise know as lingonberry). It's a tart, red, fruit related to cranberries. You will also find acerola, a red cherry-like fruit that has 30 times more vitamin C than oranges. Then we have chokeberry, an American blackberry once described as the "healthiest berry in the world". It also has apple, grape, strawberry and blueberry. (Phew – some ingredients we know!)

Although the "scientific" study wasn't done on my alternative, it will have exactly the same results. I can say that with confidence, as there has yet to be a study done on any fruit that hasn't shown a positive health effect. This is because – as corny as it sounds – all fruit has the X Factor. It is the intangible factor that nature provides to feed, heal and protect the body. The alternative ingredients I have chosen are not only closely related to the other berries and therefore without question have exactly the same health benefits, but you can actually get hold of them!

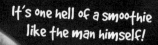

It's one hell of a smoothie like the man himself! But you don't have to wear your trousers round your armpits to drink it.

Jason's Juicy Version

30 grapes
(red or black)

1 apple
(golden delicious or apple of
your choice, make it organic it's
a super smoothie after all)

15 blueberries

9 strawberries

5 blackberries

8 cranberries
(you can juice from frozen!)

5 cherries
(pitted)

ice

Make in the same way as you
would Simon's Super Juice.

Phil "the Power" Taylor
The Big Bullseye

2 golden delicious apples
1 medium orange
1 small raw beetroot
1 medium carrot
½ medium lemon (peeled)

This is an easy and quick juice, you've just got to juice the lots and pour into a nice tall glass with plenty of deliciously cold ice.

It's the perfect juice for a hot day.

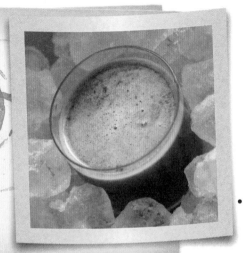

It's 180 delicious

I had the pleasure of meeting Phil *"the power"* Taylor at Juicy Oasis, boutique spa, juicing and yoga retreat in sunny Portugal. It's not often you get to say you shared a juice with a man who had won 200 professional tournaments, including 76 major titles, and a record 14 World Championships, but I was lucky enough to do so. And even though I was convinced I might give him a run for his money when playing him at darts, I think the guests can vouch the game was thoroughly entertaining at least!

It's not often you get to say you shared a juice with a man who had won 200 professional tournaments

Phil is not just a true master of the game of darts, he's also passionate about juicing and all the healthy benefits he has experienced since he started juicing. Commenting on his week at Juicy Oasis Phil had his to say "you added 20 years to my life and 10 years to my playing career".

Phil is not just a true master of the game of darts, he's also passionate about juicing

Phil has kindly offered his favourite recipe to be added to the Funky Juice Book. This recipe is *truly scrumptious* and perfect for a hot summers day! It combines the perfect combination of fruits and vegetables, proving that juice isn't all about the fruit and doesn't have to taste terrible to be good for you. I think you've hit the bullseye with this juice Phil (I know... too punny!).

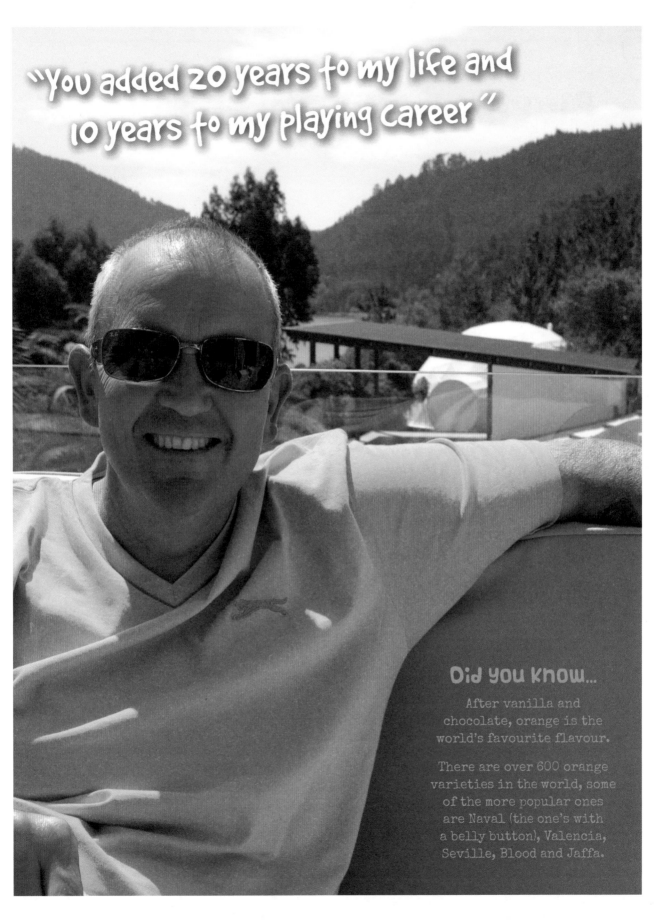

"You added 20 years to my life and 10 years to my playing career"

Did you know...

After vanilla and chocolate, orange is the world's favourite flavour.

There are over 600 orange varieties in the world, some of the more popular ones are Naval (the one's with a belly button), Valencia, Seville, Blood and Jaffa.

Linda Barker
Blueberry Breakfast Blitz

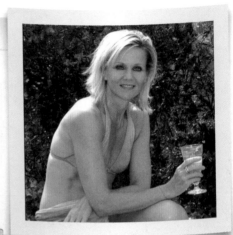

2 large handfuls blueberries
1 golden delicious apple
¼ lime

Juice the lime and apple, then blend with the blueberries. To make this into a more substantial breakfast add a tablespoon of plain natural yogurt and a tablespoon of oatmeal to the blender.

Hi, Linda Barker here. If you haven't heard about Jason Vale yet then you're in for a treat. Not only are Jason's recipes totally divine, they are phenomenally healthy. If you start to take juicing seriously you will soon notice the benefits of drinking these nutrient packed, power elixirs: better concentration, good skin, increased energy level - what's not to like? It's never been so easy to be at your very best.

"Jason, your energy and charisma was as infectious as the juice"

A year into the juicing lifestyle and I know that following one of Jason's sensible juicing plans will get me on track to tackle a heavy workload - or to feel my very best before a holiday - or quite simply when I want to be running at 100%. Watch out though - feel-ing this good is addictive!

No Need To Feel Blue In The Morning With Blueberries

Jason Vale introduced me to my new best friend, the Blueberry Breakfast Blitz, and now we meet every morning. When I want to feel great, I just head for the juicer!

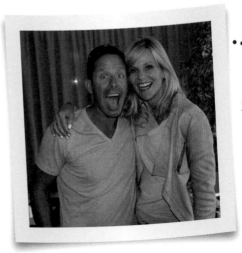

At the Juicy oa[...] Boutique Hotel a[...] Spa in Portuga[...] a blissful wee[...] of juice, yoga and rechargin[...] the spirit.

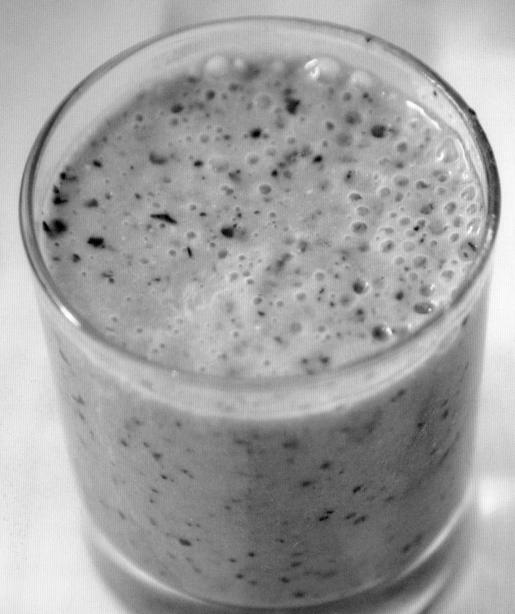

"My favourite Jason juice is the one with a quarter pineapple, one apple, a quarter cucumber or courgette/zucchini and a stick of celery – all blended with a quarter avocado, ice and a half teaspoon of spirulina."

"Juice has filtered into my brain cells quite literally and I find myself unable to get off the stuff!"

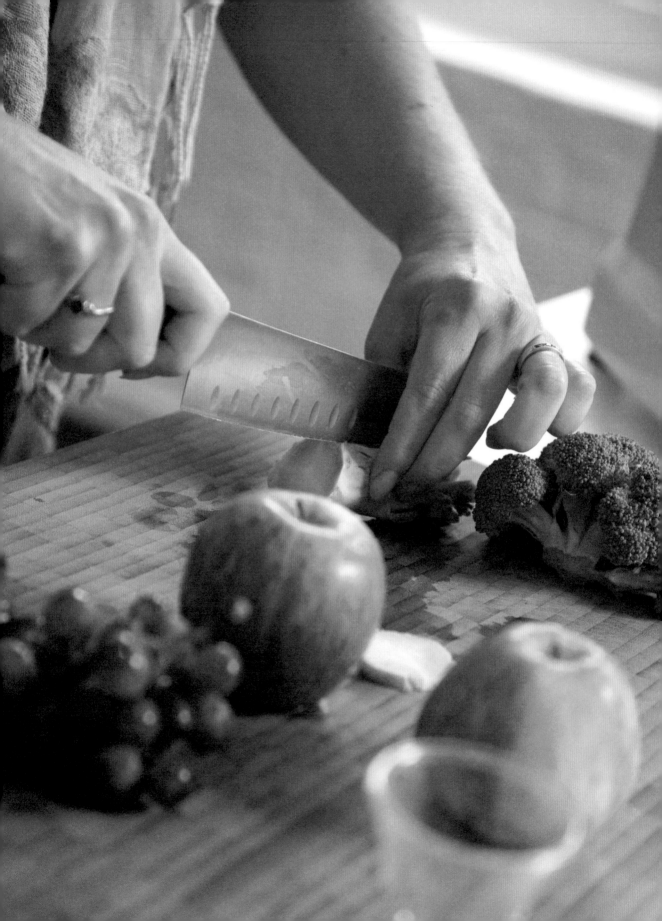

Our Juicy Community

Over the years I have been blessed to receive thousands of positive emails, letters and cards from just about every inch of the world. Many take the time to tell me their inspirational stories of how juicing has changed their lives. In this section I have included just a tiny handful from our "Juicy Community" who are helping to spread the juicy word through their own uplifting stories and their own wonderful creations.

I hope their stories, and juices, inspire you further to a healthier lifestyle and who knows – one day you may find yourself in the book!

It's A Juicy Revolution

I have also rather cheekily added myself to this section as I feel after losing so much weight, clearing my skin of psoriasis, getting rid of my asthma, stopping smoking and drinking, I should be part of this section. I am also very much part of this juicy community :) I have added my "fave" recipe in here too - hope you love it.

"Dear Jason, Having not seen my twenty four year old son for a few weeks I was struck by how glowingly well he looked. When he told me he'd read Jason's Slim For Life book and started juicing I bought it....I can hardly believe the immediate difference I felt when I started juicing daily. My bloated stomach (due to IBS) is gone, my energy levels are up, I feel in better form consistently and the taste of everything I eat is greatly enhanced. ...it just makes so much sense - humans are designed to thrive on this type of diet and so few do. Thank you."
– Antionette

"My husband and I are very much enjoying drinking delicious juices as a result of reading your books. Not only do we have more energy and better health but our hair is also going back to its original colour! We are 68 and 73 years old, so that is a wonderful surprise! Thank you"
– Audrey S

"Just thought I would drop you a very quick note to let you know how my health is improving while juicing. I have been amazed at my energy levels and the weight loss I have achieved... I am a very happy teddy xx"
– Rose

Charles Taylor's
Lean & Green

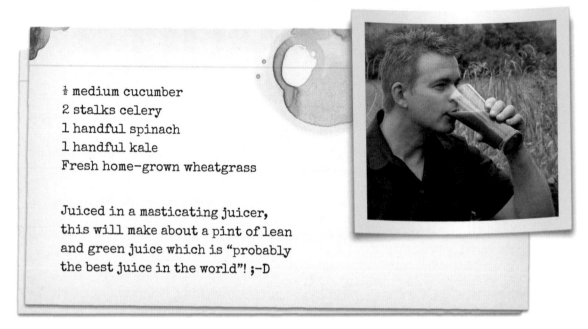

¼ medium cucumber
2 stalks celery
1 handful spinach
1 handful kale
Fresh home-grown wheatgrass

Juiced in a masticating juicer, this will make about a pint of lean and green juice which is "probably the best juice in the world"! ;-D

Juicing came about from the quest for a healthier lifestyle. I initially tested my pH which frightened the life out of me! I became overwhelmed with lots of books that contained scientific data, which started to confuse me.

A friend lent me *Turbo Charge your Life* by Jason Vale. Then I bought another of Jason's books *Kick the Drink Easily* and haven't had alcohol since – I now only drink when I am sober! Jason's philosophy resonated in my mind & made sense! I was finally on the road to health and vitality!

I'm Finally Off The Junk-Food Treadmill

I feel incredible! I've lost a remarkable amount of weight – 4 stone (25 kg / 55 lbs) in 4 months! I sleep less, eat less, and I'm finally off the junk-food treadmill. My wife can't keep her hands off me! I no longer look or act my age! At work, my clarity is incredible. My performance, efficiency and job rates have improved. It is no longer about the weight I lost – I am healthier and happier then I could ever have imagined.

I Mostly Stick To Vegetables Because They Are Easier To Grow In The Uk

I tend to stick to more vegetable based juices rather than fruit. Vegetables are easier to grow in the UK than fruit. Daily I will have the Lean & Green juice. I might add some broccoli, beetroot, mint, ginger or whatever else I might have. That's what I love about juicing, if you can't make the mix because you've run out of something you can normally create something else.

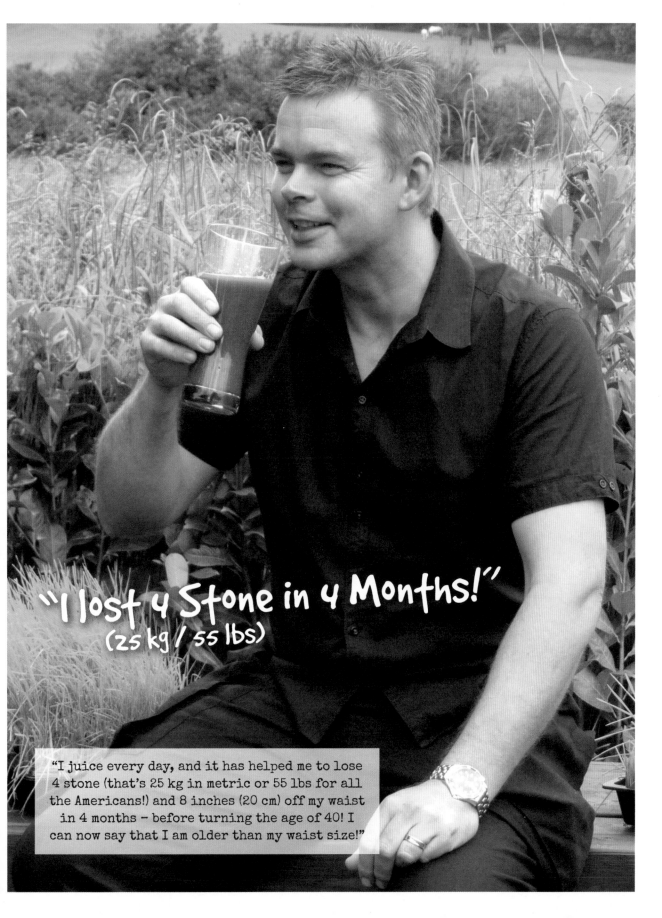

"I lost 4 Stone in 4 Months!"
(25 kg / 55 lbs)

"I juice every day, and it has helped me to lose 4 stone (that's 25 kg in metric or 55 lbs for all the Americans!) and 8 inches (20 cm) off my waist in 4 months – before turning the age of 40! I can now say that I am older than my waist size!"

Ken Howlett's
Fruity Filler

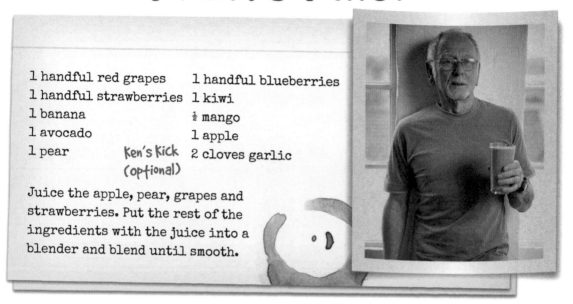

1 handful red grapes   1 handful blueberries
1 handful strawberries   1 kiwi
1 banana   ½ mango
1 avocado   1 apple
1 pear   Ken's Kick 2 cloves garlic
                (optional)

Juice the apple, pear, grapes and strawberries. Put the rest of the ingredients with the juice into a blender and blend until smooth.

I'm Ken and I'm a level 2 gym instructor running a gym for the over 50s. I'm "A1" fit and the quality of my life is great at the age of 75! I'm active and take good care of myself. I certainly don't feel my age in mind, body or spirit.

It's Never Too Late To Take Care of Your Health

You might not think it but up until the age of 45 I drank, smoked, ate all the wrong food and didn't exercise at all.

Then "Eureka"!! I got fed up of feeling older than my years and decided to turn it around. So I stopped smoking and drinking and joined an athletics club where I started running. I also started eating what my body needed – you know, the healthy stuff. It took a little time, and initially a lot of effort, but once I started to feel the benefits of a healthier and more active lifestyle I knew I

could never go back to how I was.

Within 18 months of starting running I'd run my first London Marathon! I've run 5 now, 5 Great North Runs and numerous other races. I coached athletics for 12 years as a UKA level 2 endurance coach and ran circuit training sessions weekly, sharing with others the message that it's never too late to start. Health and fitness is well worth the effort of obtaining and keeping.

Try "Ken's Kick" – If You Dare!

Juices and smoothies form a very important part of my fitness regime. I have smoothies everyday and they're always full of fruits, vegetables, seeds, essential oils and my favourite ingredient – garlic! I call it "Ken's Kick". Some may say garlic is a bit strong – but I think it gives my smoothies and wonderful health boost and a great creamy taste. Try it if you dare!

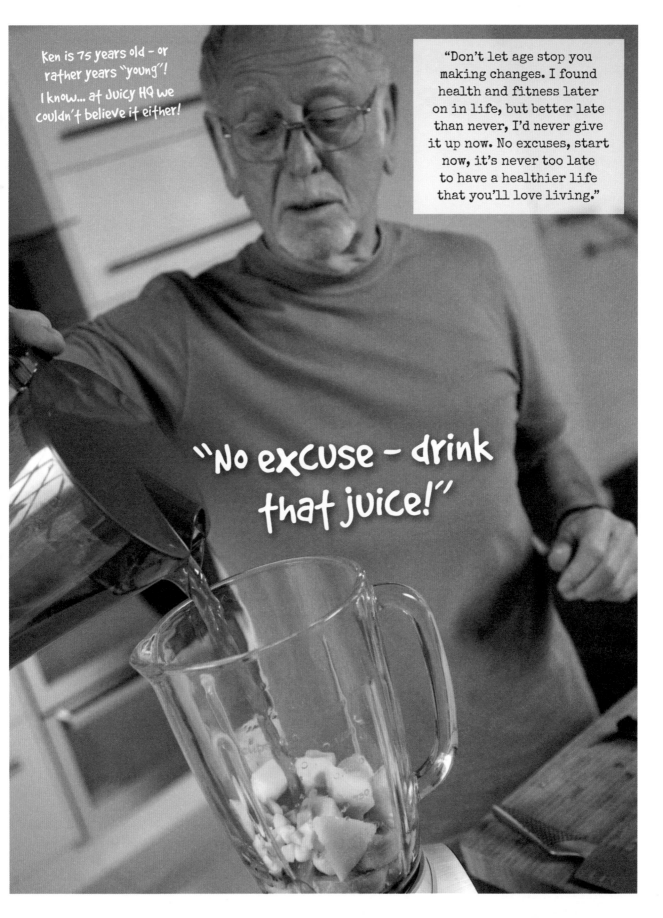

Anita Lewis's Brilliant Breakfast Smoothie

2 apples
1 banana
1 handful fresh parsley
3 Tbsp date syrup — *or 4 whole dates*
ice *optional*

Juice the apples. Add the juice and everything else into a blender, then whizz it all up – simple! Add ice cubes if you want a nice, refreshing wake-up call.

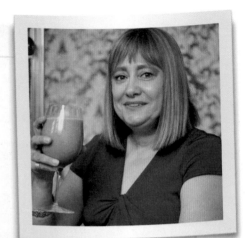

Forty years ago people thought that eating raw carrots, salads and lentils was eccentric – strange even! Some people still think that way. I don't though, I've been attracted to this way of eating for most of my life, despite the lack of support I received in those early days. In the late 1970s I tried to buy a juicer – but in those days juicers were very slow, difficult to clean and you had to cut everything up to juice it! I'm so pleased that juicing has moved along since then. It's a lot easier now to not only juice but buy a wide variety of fresh produce.

Juicing Helped Me With An Important Milestone

So much of the food that's easily available to us today is bad for us and void of vitamins and nutrients, it's like "plastic" food. I believe it's very important to eat a healthy diet. My father died at the age of 59, his lifestyle was not very healthy and, perhaps, if he'd made some changes to his diet he would've enjoyed a longer life. I'm 60 now and grateful (really grateful) that I've made changes and stayed healthy – reaching 60 was a milestone for me. Juicing has remained an easy way to drink lots of fruit and vegetables, you get more in a juice than you could in a meal.

A Perfect Juice For Breakfast

I love my "Brilliant Breakfast Smoothie" recipe, dates and bananas together – yum! Dates are fibre-rich, which is good for one's colon. I've always liked the taste of parsley, although you might think it's an unusual addition, I think it's a refreshing green addition that can also aid digestion. A perfect juice for breakfast.

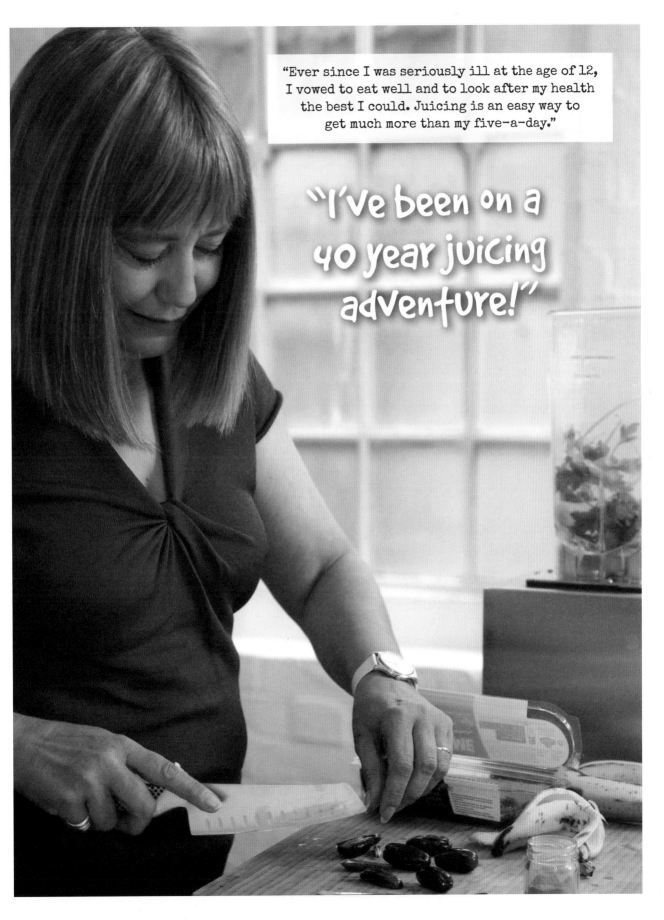

"Ever since I was seriously ill at the age of 12, I vowed to eat well and to look after my health the best I could. Juicing is an easy way to get much more than my five-a-day."

"I've been on a 40 year juicing adventure!"

Carol Brace's
Grandma's Brew

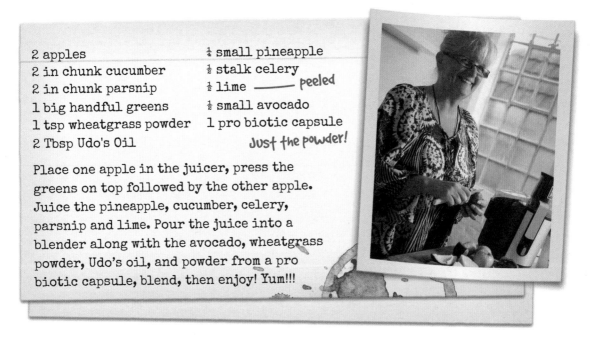

2 apples
2 in chunk cucumber
2 in chunk parsnip
1 big handful greens
1 tsp wheatgrass powder
2 Tbsp Udo's Oil

¼ small pineapple
½ stalk celery
½ lime ——— peeled
½ small avocado
1 pro biotic capsule
Just the powder!

Place one apple in the juicer, press the greens on top followed by the other apple. Juice the pineapple, cucumber, celery, parsnip and lime. Pour the juice into a blender along with the avocado, wheatgrass powder, Udo's oil, and powder from a pro biotic capsule, blend, then enjoy! Yum!!!

I was 58 years old and looking forward to retirement, my plan was to spend the next 20 years or so growing old gracefully, but this was not meant to be!

Juicing Has Given Me A New Lease of Life

I read my first book by Jason Vale: *7lbs in 7 days*. After reading it cover to cover (as the man said!) I did the detox which set me on an adventure that shows no sign of ending. 4 years later, I'm a fully qualified Juice Master Natural Juice Therapist running my own business.

I walked Hadrian's Wall In Six Days – Nearly 20 Miles A Day

I recently took a week off and walked the length of Hadrian's Wall with a friend, it took over 6 days and I enjoyed every moment of it. Would you believe we walked a total of 105 miles? I wouldn't have been able to do 5 miles in a day 4 years ago let alone nearly 20! Juicing really has given me a new lease of life.

I feel Fitter Now Than I Did 10 Years Ago

As we age our bodies begin to deteriorate, we find we cannot do the things we used to do in our youth. I feel that juicing has enabled me to slow down the ageing process. I feel younger, healthier, fitter, more alert at 62 that I did at 52. I stumbled upon juicing later in my life and although I wish I had known about it when I was younger I firmly believe that it's never to late to make positive changes to your life.

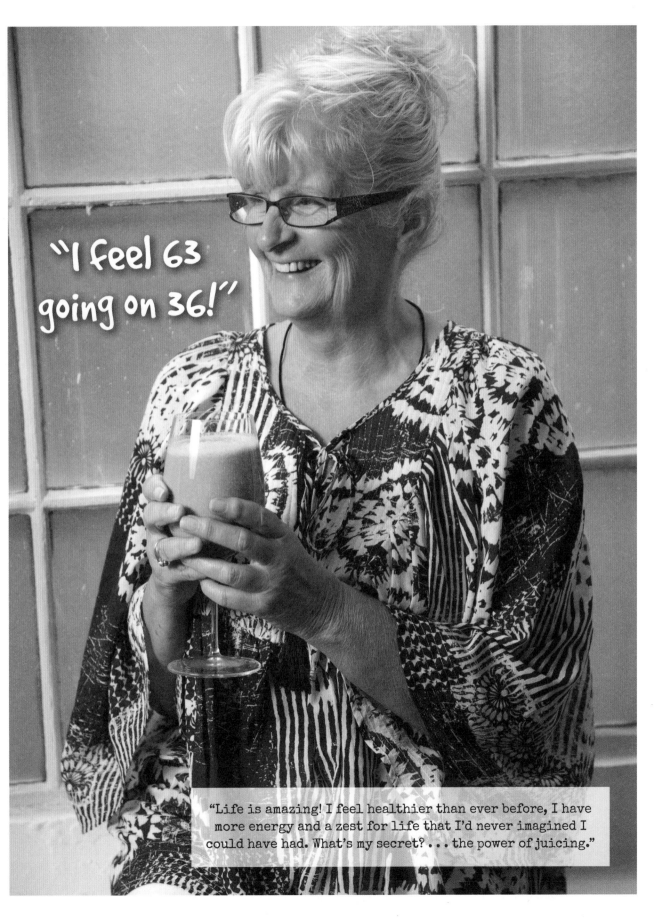

"I feel 63 going on 36!"

"Life is amazing! I feel healthier than ever before, I have more energy and a zest for life that I'd never imagined I could have had. What's my secret? . . . the power of juicing."

Debbieleigh Driver's
Avo-Coco-Cado-Nut!

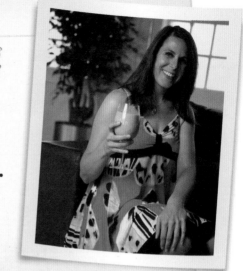

1 coconut
½ medium cucumber
¼ medium pineapple *peeled*
½ medium avocado
ice

Empty the coconut water into the blender.
Juice the pineapple and cucumber, then
add the juice with the avocado and ice
to the coconut water and blend.

I've been a vegan for more than 15 years, and although I'm very careful about what I eat, a few years ago I began to suffer from crippling IBS. The doctors prescribed me the usual pills but they didn't really ease my symptoms and they didn't fit with my philosophy on life as a vegan.

Luckily I found out about Jason "Juice Master" Vale, and I took myself off on one of his retreats in Turkey. The results were outstanding! Not only did I lose 10 lbs but my symptoms decreased and I had a huge surge in energy. IBS meant I didn't have the energy to keep going with my usual active lifestyle, so it was wonderful to feel my energy coming back again.

Juicing Did More For My IBS Than The Doctors Could

Since the diagnosis, over 2 years ago, I have detoxed at the Juice Master retreat in Turkey several times and now I have virtually no IBS symptoms. It's all thanks to juicing, in my opinion. I think it's much easier for my stomach to digest juice and I can get a lot more nutrition from a single juice than chomping on lots of food.

Juice Is Easier For My Body To Digest

Since I started juicing I've come up with loads of different recipes, it's fun to experiment with different flavours and textures. Smoothies are great and filling and juice shots are amazing for an energy boost. My favourite at the moment is the wonderful Avo-coco-cado-nut. I love to have a big glass before I go on stage and sing. The coconut is hydrating and leaves me feeling awake and focused, and the avocado is fantastic for the skin. It's filling, and most of all it tastes refreshingly great.

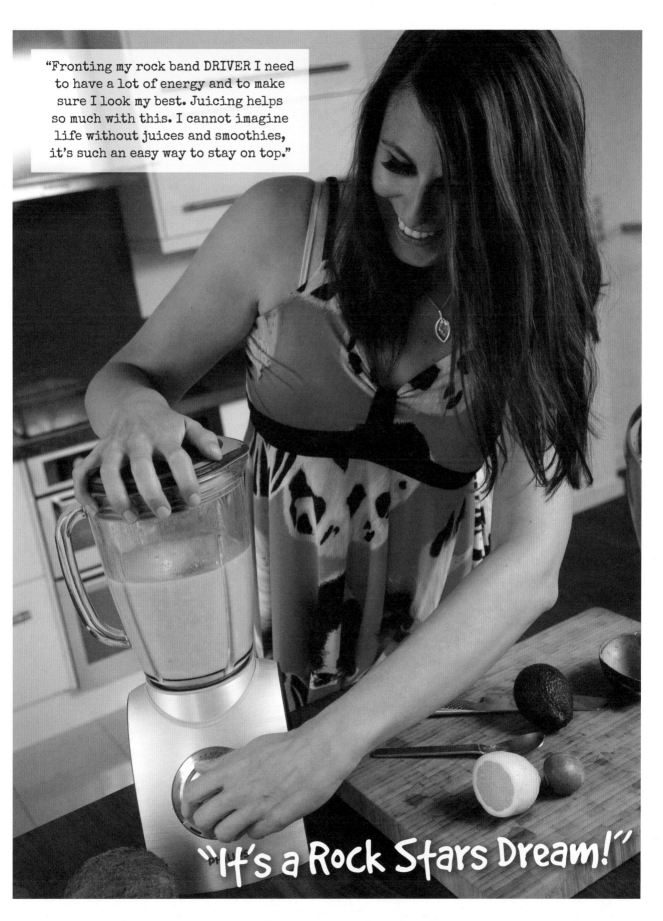

"Fronting my rock band DRIVER I need to have a lot of energy and to make sure I look my best. Juicing helps so much with this. I cannot imagine life without juices and smoothies, it's such an easy way to stay on top."

"It's a Rock Stars Dream!"

Kevin Doyle's
Cashew Strength

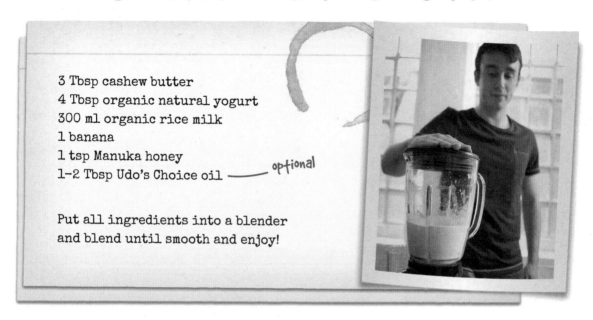

3 Tbsp cashew butter
4 Tbsp organic natural yogurt
300 ml organic rice milk
1 banana
1 tsp Manuka honey
1-2 Tbsp Udo's Choice oil —— optional

Put all ingredients into a blender
and blend until smooth and enjoy!

I got into juicing a couple of years ago when I read one of the Juice Master books. Juicing's great, I can get live nutrients into my body. A good wholesome diet and staying fit and active is great for mind, body and soul.

It's been really easy for me to get into juicing, although some of my mates are a bit bemused by it! I remember walking down the road with a pineapple in my hand and my mate from my football team asked me "What the hell are you going to do with that?" and I said "Juice it!". The look on his face was priceless!

I Make Juices & Smoothies To Stay In Peak Condition

I love keeping fit. I lift weights 3 times a week and play Gaelic Football for my local team in Dublin. I make juices and smoothies to stay in peak condition for playing games and just for general fitness.

Cashew Strength is my favourite – of course! It's the perfect blend of goodness after the gym or a training session! The cashew butter is packed with protein and contains phosphorus, magnesium, iron and zinc which are important for muscle growth. Not only does rice milk have a glorious flavour, it also contains fat soluble vitamins A, D, B, calcium and iron. The natural organic yogurt has the pro biotic cultures for healthy digestion. The good old banana can't be left out of a sports smoothie, it contains the important mineral potassium that replaces the electrolytes lost through sweat during a workout. And Manuka honey is an essential ingredient due to its healing properties. What a nutrient dense gem of a muscle building smoothie and most importantly it tastes great!

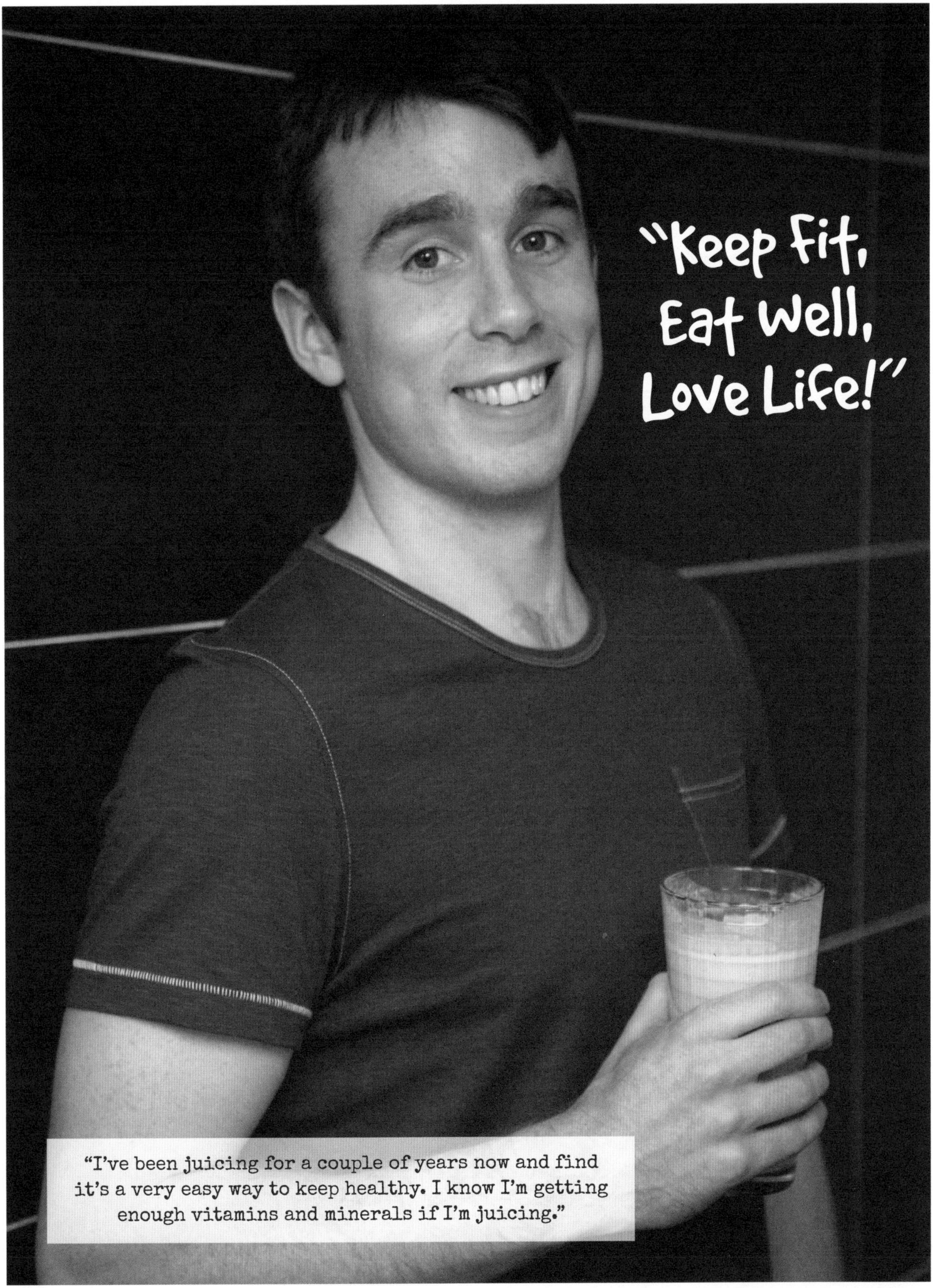

"Keep Fit,
Eat Well,
Love Life!"

"I've been juicing for a couple of years now and find it's a very easy way to keep healthy. I know I'm getting enough vitamins and minerals if I'm juicing."

Irene Fitzmaurice's
Pineapple Delite

10 medium oranges
1 lemon
2 grapefruit
1 medium pineapple
3 bananas
1 cm chunk ginger —— *to taste*

Peel the oranges and lemon leaving on the pith. Juice the pineapple and citrus fruit (and ginger if you like it) then put the juice into a blender with 3 bananas and blend until smooth. Delicious!

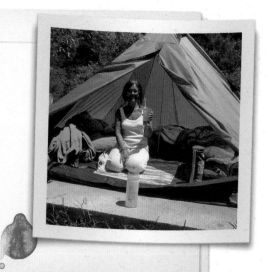

I've always had problems with my weight and spent a lot of time struggling to shift my *excess baggage*, so to speak. I was 4 ft 10 (177 cm) and weighed nearly 12 stone (76 kg / 168 lbs), I felt like Mrs Blobby! I knew I wanted to be thinner and healthier but I was never really motivated enough to do it.

I Struggled With My Weight & I Felt Like Mrs Blobby

When I turned 60, I took the jump – literally! I did a parachute jump to celebrate this momentous milestone, but I needed to lose a few pounds before I could do it – that was my incentive! I started juicing and not only lost the weight, but more than that – I felt full of energy and vitality.

The jump was fantastic, it was like flying without wings. It was an experience I will always remember and juicing helped me to take that plunge and change my life.

I Practically Live At The Juice Master Retreats

Juicing is incredible! I can't get enough of it! I love the way it makes me feel – healthy and full of life. It's like I have this ball of sunshine and happiness inside me, I feel so happy that I just love everybody and want to spread the sunshine around.

And a big bonus now is I don't have to worry about loosing weight, I have and it's stayed off this time. I'm a light and happy 8½ stone (54 kg / 119 lbs)!

Don't Waste Time – Change Your Life Forever!

Why waste time wanting change but not making it? Or worrying about it and never feeling happy? Don't think about it! Do it! Change your life forever – I did!

"Jason is my hero I will never be able to thank him enough for showing me how to get out of, and more importantly stay out of, the food trap. I will love him forever."

"I took the jump & changed my life!"

Jacqueline Huismans'
Tropical Juice

5 large oranges
2 bananas
1 Tbsp grated coconut
1 handful ice

Juice the oranges (peeled).
Place everything else in the
blender and blend until smooth.
Easy and incredibly tasty!

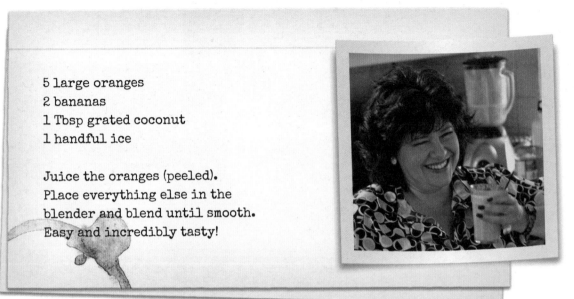

I've never really liked fruit. I like the taste of apples, but their flesh and skin – not so much. I like bananas, but only if I'm really in the mood for one; and other fruit doesn't fare too well with me either! As a result I hardly eat any fruit. But as I've been getting older, I've been thinking more about my health; and I started thinking that perhaps my aversion to fruit needed addressing.

I Needed To Watch My Diet, But I've Never Liked Fruit

I pondered on the matter for a while, then I noticed an advert for a juicer and it just hit me – this is it! I don't need to *eat* fruit. I can live healthily by *drinking* fresh fruit juice instead! So I surfed the net, found the Juice Master's site and became even more enthusiastic! I never knew that there are juicers that could take whole apples and handle fruits with tough skins, like pineapple. I was thrilled to find that it would be really easy to get into juicing. This marked the start of a new, fruitier lifestyle. I bought a juicer and loads of fruit and started juicing and juicing and juicing!

I Realized I Didn't Need To Eat Fruit – I Could Drink It!

I experiment whenever I can and don't follow recipes so much anymore. Almost any combination tastes great, so whatever fruit is around I'll juice or blend it into something heavenly.

Lately I've been buying some frozen fruit to blend with fresh juice. Blueberries, raspberries, mango, tropical mixes – it's like using little fruity ice-cubes to make my juices refreshingly cool!

"why eat fruit when you can juice it?"

Mark Locke
The Blood Transfusion

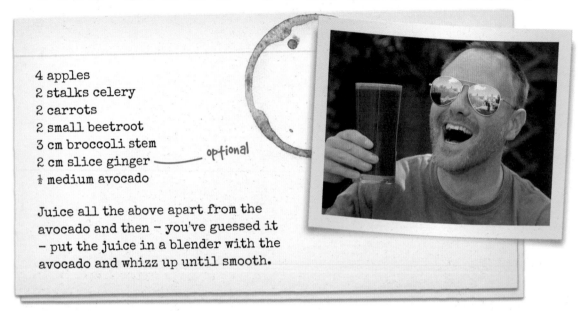

4 apples
2 stalks celery
2 carrots
2 small beetroot
3 cm broccoli stem
2 cm slice ginger —— optional
½ medium avocado

Juice all the above apart from the
avocado and then – you've guessed it
– put the juice in a blender with the
avocado and whizz up until smooth.

I was overweight in my 20s but my 30s were a different story and juicing played a big part in keeping me trim and healthy. Last summer I wrote and directed a film – a comedy no less! It was a very busy time and I lost my way a bit, food wise. I took the "easy" option of eating whatever was there – lots of "stodgy" food and sugary snacks – and I put weight on fast!

I HAD To Fit Into Those Spandex Trousers for My Mum's 70th

After the summer I knew I had to lose the weight from all that junk and snack food, especially as I was having a big party with my Mum to celebrate my 40th and her 70th – a big milestone for both of us. The theme was "Rock 'n' Roll" which would involve me wearing some rather tight spandex trousers. As you can appreciate I really didn't want to be overweight wearing those!

With only a week to go I did Jason's *7lbs in 7 days* Juice Master diet. I stuck to it religiously, including the work-outs. To begin with it was tough. But by day three I started to have loads more energy and felt lighter on my feet. By day five I could literally feel my body changing shape! It's weird what you crave when you're doing the *7lbs* program, you'd expect to be craving unhealthy stuff but what I was really dying for was a big salad or some nice homemade soup!

It's Easier Than You Think To Get Back on Track

I lost a whopping 12 lbs, I fitted into my spandex and had a great party! I haven't piled the weight back on after either. Busy summers and bad food reminded me that it's really important to take care of your health but also that if you do slip up it's easier than you think to get back on track.

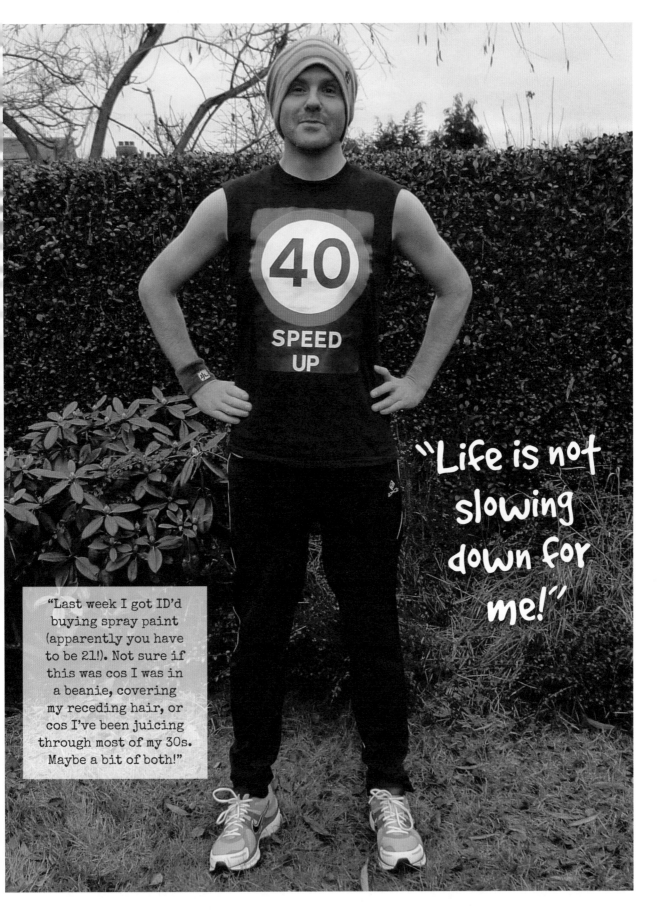

40

SPEED UP

"Life is not slowing down for me!"

"Last week I got ID'd buying spray paint (apparently you have to be 21!). Not sure if this was cos I was in a beanie, covering my receding hair, or cos I've been juicing through most of my 30s. Maybe a bit of both!"

Polly Noble's
Knight in Shining Greenery!

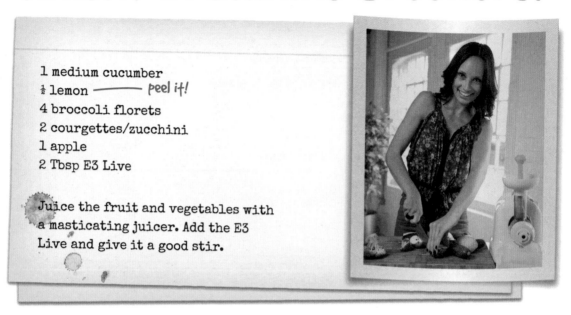

1 medium cucumber
½ lemon ——— peel it!
4 broccoli florets
2 courgettes/zucchini
1 apple
2 Tbsp E3 Live

Juice the fruit and vegetables with a masticating juicer. Add the E3 Live and give it a good stir.

Hi, I'm Polly, I'm a holistic health and raw food coach, inspirational speaker and author. I'm on a healing mission. Being diagnosed with cancer for the first time aged just 24 ignited a deep desire to help my body heal. I began juicing while undergoing simultaneous chemo and radiotherapy as a way to flood my body with much needed vitamins, minerals, phytonutrients and oxygen.

Four years later I was told my cancer had returned and was incurable. I was offered radiotherapy as a palliative treatment but having suffered so badly with side-effects the first time I said "No thanks!" It just felt like an incredibly disempowering stance to take with the odds of success being so low. From that moment on I embarked on a cancer butt-kicking mission using juicing, amongst other things, to give my body the best chance of creating optimum health.

I'm on A Cancer Butt-Kicking Mission Using Juicing

My juices started out as fruit combos but I like to keep my sugar consumption to a minimum so I'm now a fully-fledged green juice junkie. I love, *love*, **love** green juice. It's my daily staple, my best friend, my saviour – literally! I take it everywhere I go: on the tube, in the car and even to meetings which raises a few eyebrows! The chlorophyll and phytonutrients from green leafy vegetables help to boost my immune system, cleanse my liver and keep me feeling truly alive and well. I can safely say as far as best friends go, you can't get better than green juice. It will be with me for life – which, by the way, I plan on living for a very long time!

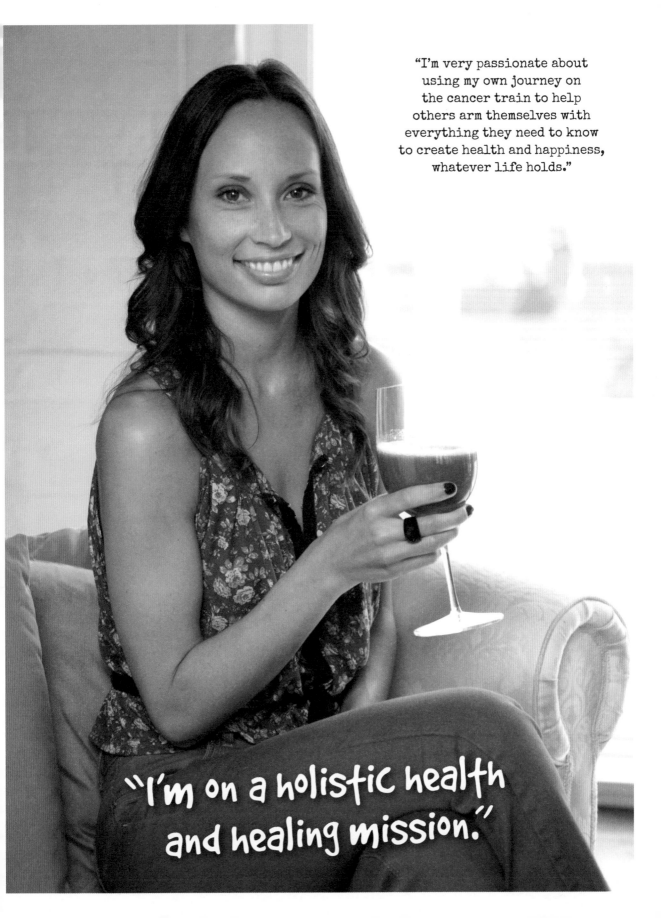

"I'm very passionate about using my own journey on the cancer train to help others arm themselves with everything they need to know to create health and happiness, whatever life holds."

"I'm on a holistic health and healing mission."

Shaun Chiole's
Diplomatic Immunity

2 apples

1 inch beetroot

1 handful baby spinach

1 large carrot

1 handful raspberries

2 brazil nuts

1 inch pineapple

1 inch broccoli stem

1 handful watercress

½ lime — *peeled*

½ avocado

Juice it all apart from the avocado and the nuts – you'll need to blend those into the juice after.

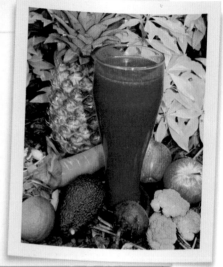

Being of slim build and good health, I'd lived life without thinking much about what I put in my mouth. So I was surprised when, in 2010, I developed a bad case of digestive issues and acid reflux. After playing doctor ping-pong and being a blood-test pin cushion, I finished up with a proton pump inhibitor which didn't really work, in fact it caused my white blood cell to drop. I've always been fit and healthy, so the loss of energy and the pain was a wake-up call.

The Loss of Energy & Pain Was A Wake-Up Call

Colleagues at work were supportive and recommended wheatgrass and juicing. So I found Jason Vale and started juicing my way back to health. My first juice was *The Ultimate Health Boost Juice*, it was a bizarre concoction of fruit and veg – what on earth would it taste like?! One gulp later and I don't think I stopped grinning all evening!

Both my wife and I were instantly converted – for life – literally! We began juicing every single day. I wish I'd known about juicing earlier in my life, but it's never too late to start and my children will have the benefit and enjoyment of juicing for life!

One Gulp & I Was Converted To Juicing

Diplomatic Immunity is a great antibacterial, blood builder that boosts and maintains the thymus – the commanding officer of the immune system army. This blend of very powerful antioxidants and phytonutrients fights antigens in the blood, gut and mucous membranes. It also contains the top 10 minerals and vitamins that are crucial for improving immunity. And who says everything that's good for you tastes bad? This juice has a silky texture and gorgeous flavour, I cannot get enough of this juice. It is staggering that something so delicious is so good for you.

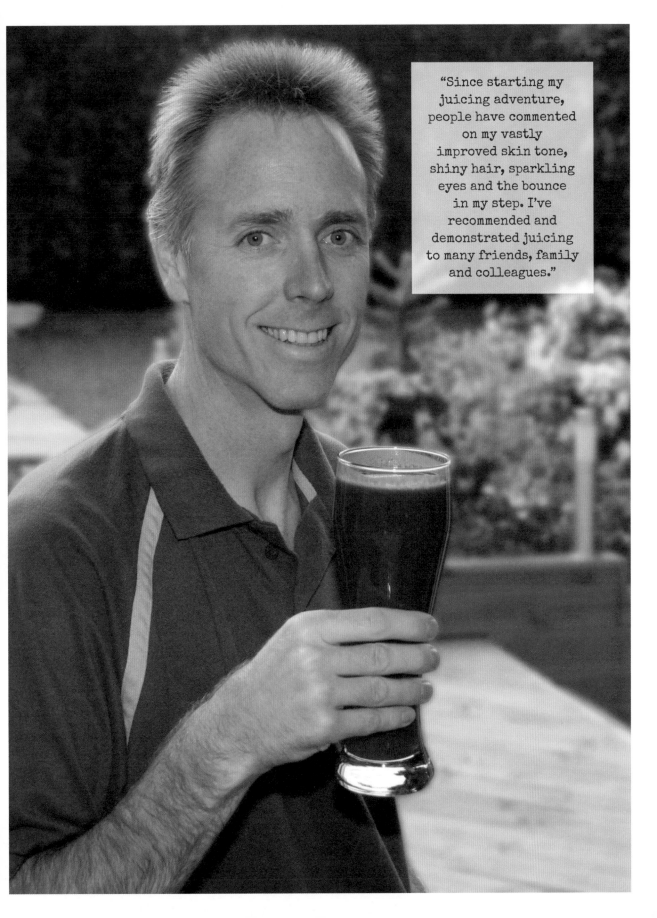

"Since starting my juicing adventure, people have commented on my vastly improved skin tone, shiny hair, sparkling eyes and the bounce in my step. I've recommended and demonstrated juicing to many friends, family and colleagues."

Sybille Muir's
Avocanana Rocks!

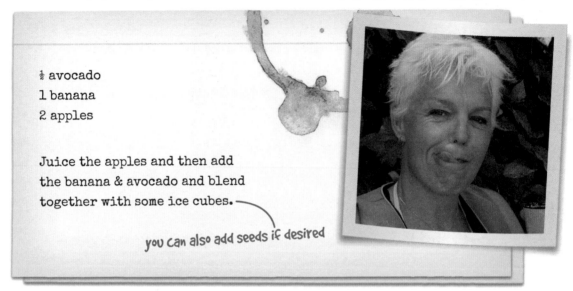

¼ avocado
1 banana
2 apples

Juice the apples and then add
the banana & avocado and blend
together with some ice cubes.

you can also add seeds if desired

Guten tag! I'm a 51 year old German Account Manager for an IT company. I live a very active lifestyle in Scotland. I've always been an active person and enjoyed doing all kinds of sports; but I tended to comfort eat, so I was always a little heavier than I wanted to be (with a bit of a muffin top). I know many ladies have similar issues.

I'm Active & Enjoy Sports, But Struggled With My Muffin Top

I then discovered Jason and his philosophy on diet and health, and I was hooked from day one! It completely changed my life and the way I viewed food. I L-O-V-E to eat, juice, and make smoothies – all from Jason's recipes. It's all natural and good for me. No more eating for comfort – I don't need to! I don't crave bad foods anymore, just the wholesome good foods. And I haven't had anymore problems with weight – in fact I don't ever think about it now because I feel

so fit, happy, energized and confident!

With my new lease of life, I took the bull by the horns, and became a contestant on *Total Wipeout*. I spent a week in Argentina competing with 19 (much younger) contestants. And I did well! I came 6th during the qualifier. Those big red balls can't stop me!

With My New Lease of Life I Became A Contestant on Total Wipeout

I'm active almost everyday – skiing, swimming, cycling, yoga, scuba diving – and I teach Callanetics. All this and I have a very demanding job that involves lots of travel. But with a juice or smoothie by my side, it doesn't daunt me at all!

"Avocanana Rocks!" is my favourite. I have it for breakfast or after my exercise session or any other time during the day when I need something "substantial" to keep me going for the next couple of hours!

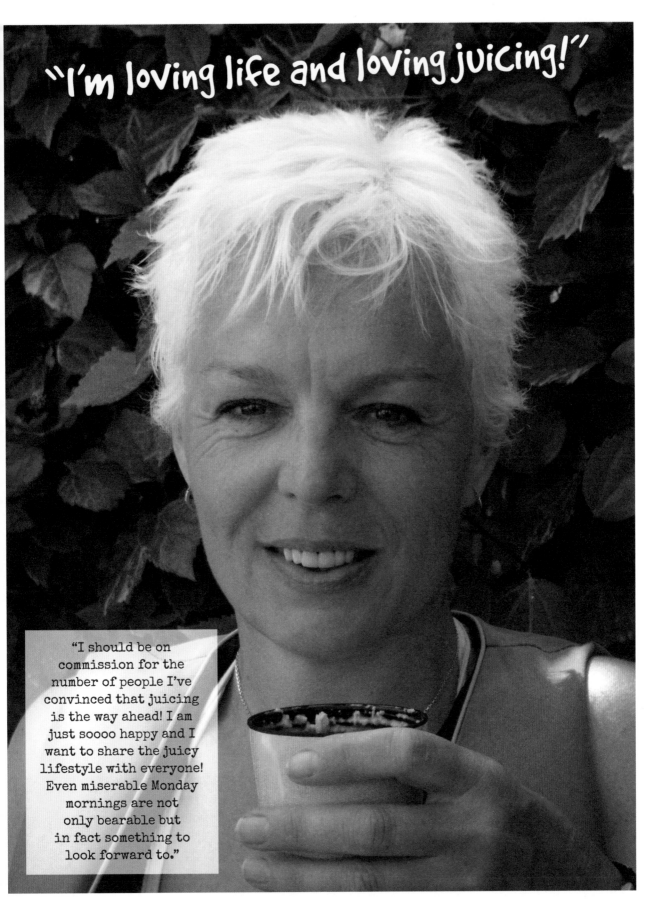

"I'm loving life and loving juicing!"

"I should be on commission for the number of people I've convinced that juicing is the way ahead! I am just soooo happy and I want to share the juicy lifestyle with everyone! Even miserable Monday mornings are not only bearable but in fact something to look forward to."

Stuart Sharp's
Protein Power Boost

3 apples   3 carrots
1 in chunk ginger   ½ avocado
2 Tbsp Juice Master hemp protein powder
1 tsp Juice Master Spirulina Powder
½ tsp Juice Master Wheatgrass Powder

Juice the apples, carrots and ginger.
Pour into a blender and add the
avocado, protein powder, spirulina
and wheatgrass. Blend until smooth.

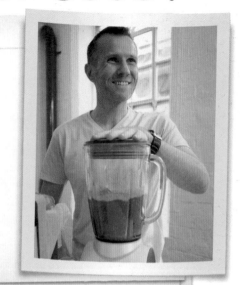

I was actually inspired by my twin brother (not identical, if you're wondering). He returned home from university looking extremely vibrant and radiating loads of positive energy. As you can imagine I wanted to share in this new found health and vitality – what did I have to do? His secret was drinking freshly extracted fruit and vegetable juices – not from cartons or bottles, but the real thing. I guess you could call it "home-made" juice – the good stuff!

I Was Inspired By My Twin Brother

Through his shining example he imbued in me his passion for juicing and living a healthy and nutritious lifestyle.

That was 15 years ago and I haven't stopped juicing in all that time. I never feel more alive and energetic than when I'm drinking freshly extracted juice, it's a fundamental part of my daily routine – I just love it!

My absolute favourite is Jason's Turbo Charge Smoothie – the meal in a glass . . . but that's a recipe from another book!

Juicing Is Essential For Losing Those Last Few ounces of fat

I'm very 'into' my own personal fitness and I exercise to the extreme!! When I'm training particularly hard, juicing is essential for loosing those last few ounces of body fat. It's also crucial for giving my body those all important vital nutrients.

Particularly important for me is my post-workout recovery drink. That's when the body is primed to absorb nutrients, especially protein, so my "Protein Power Boost" juice helps me do just that. *Juice Master's Hemp Protein Powder* is my powder of choice as it is a complete, nondairy plant protein that contains all the essential amino acids and the biologically active protein edestin.

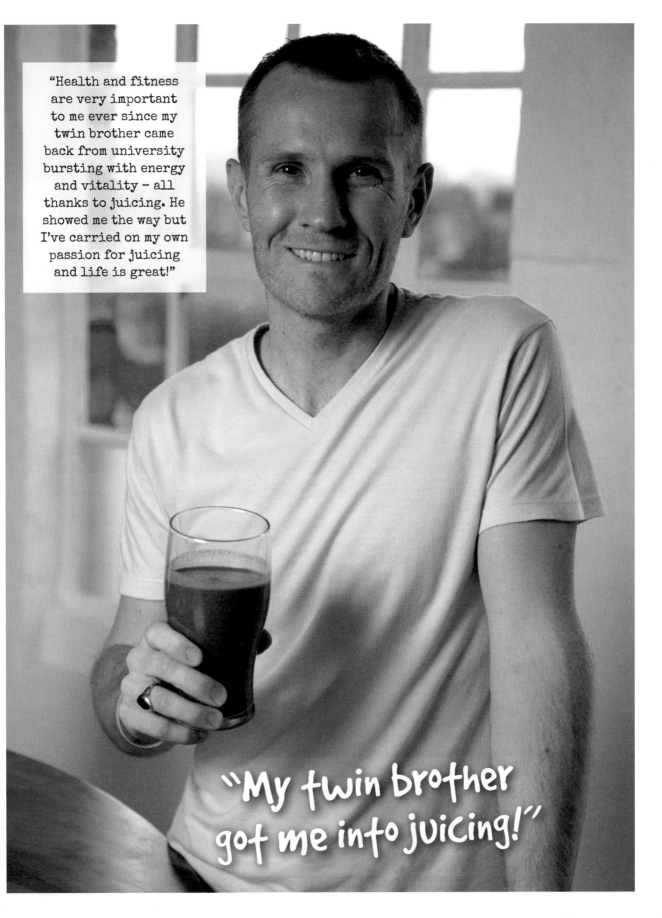

"Health and fitness are very important to me ever since my twin brother came back from university bursting with energy and vitality – all thanks to juicing. He showed me the way but I've carried on my own passion for juicing and life is great!"

"My twin brother got me into juicing!"

Verity Spencer-Sewell's
Good Life, Green Life

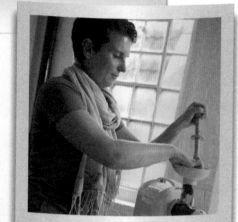

12–15 red seedless grapes   1 handful watercress
1 large broccoli floret   1 in broccoli stem
2 "chutefuls" wheatgrass   2 apples
use wheatgrass powder if not using a masticating juicer

Centrifugal Juicer: Put one apple into the chute followed by the watercress then sandwich with the other apple. Turn on machine. Juice broccoli, grapes then add wheatgrass powder and blend or really, really stir!

Masticating Juicer: Simply juice all the ingredients together!

I started juicing last summer after being diagnosed with primary & secondary breast cancer at age 37. A good friend told me about juicing and the Juice Master, she recommended getting *Keep it Simple* by Jason Vale and a Phillips Aluminium juicer so that I could have healthy juices at tough times like Chemotherapy. While other patients recovered from their treatments with chips, crisps and chocolate bars, I was fortunate enough to be drinking live juices and smoothies that gave my body vital vitamins and minerals. I cannot imagine doing it any other way – it's part of my life, for good.

Juicing Helped Me Get Through Chemotherapy

Friends and family that come to visit or stay are always keen to know what juice I will be serving up after breakfast: they look forward to their health kick. I recently upgraded to a masticating juicer so I could extract more juice from the vegetables and fruit and I can also juice fresh wheatgrass. One friend calls my juicer the "*Wallace & Gromit-erator*"!

I've tried many recipes from Jason's book, but now I mostly freestyle and juice whatever is in the fridge – within reason!

Juicing Is A Great Way To Give Myself The Best Nutrition

The ingredients for "Good Life, Green Life" and most of my juices are all to fight my cancer and give my body the best nutrition. They keep me, my husband, and daughter India feeling healthy and vitalized.

I juice every day and combine my juices with fresh organic food, including sprouting mung beans, chickpeas, alfalfa and – of course – we also grow our own wheatgrass on the windowsill.

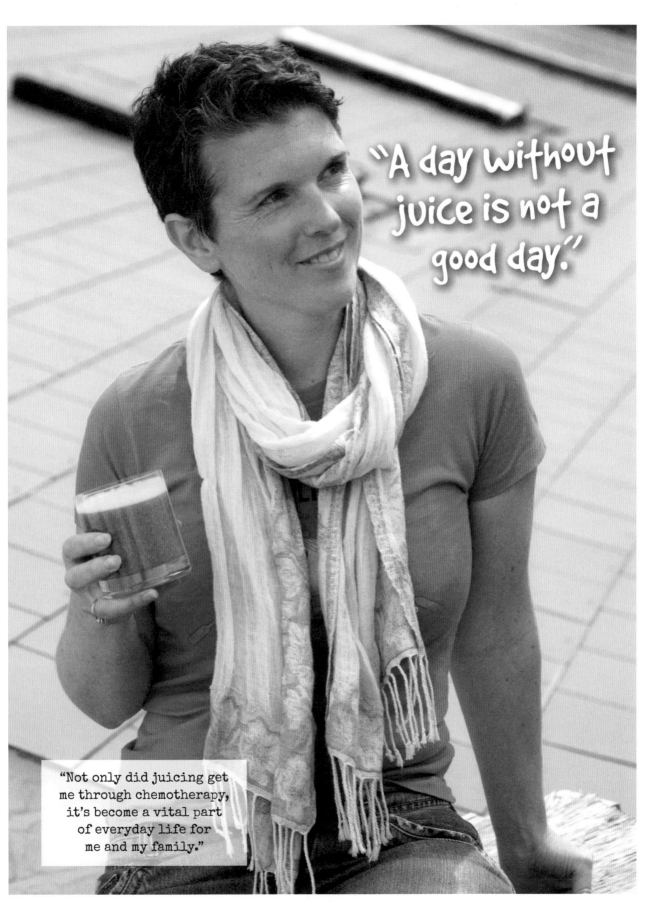

"A day without juice is not a good day."

"Not only did juicing get me through chemotherapy, it's become a vital part of everyday life for me and my family."

Olive MacDonagh's
Loop d' Loop

2 apples
1 handful spinach
¼ courgette/zucchini
¼ lime

½ medium cucumber
¼ avocado
¼ lemon
Lots of ice

Juice the apples, spinach, cucumber, courgette / zucchini, lemon and lime (don't peel the lemon or lime for extra zing!)

Put the avocado and ice into a blender and add the juice. Whisk until smooth!

For variety you can add a carrot or a couple of stalks of celery and it still tastes grrrrrrrrrrreat!

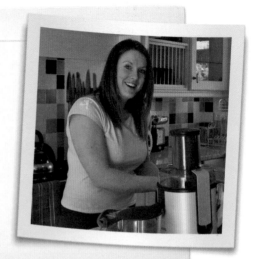

I got into juicing a couple of years ago after being quite ill. At the time I was working in a stressful job and not looking after my diet. I was diagnosed with stage IV endometriosis and ovarian cysts, and had two serious operations. I was confined to bed (or couch) for weeks-on-end when recovering. I started researching online about natural alternatives to help healing. Then at a health seminar in Dublin I heard about juicing and was keen to check it out.

Juicing Helped Me To Recover From Two Serious operations

I bought a juicer, it included Jason's *7lbs in 7 Days* book. After trying lots of different juices I inspired a rugby friend to get a juicer and do the book's 7 day juicing plan with me. Word spread about how great we were feeling (girls like to chat!). Since then lots of the rugby girls have started juicing

for energy and performance. I even went to Turkey to the 7 day retreat with another friend and we absolutely loved it! "Best holiday of our lives" we both said.

Now I'm Getting Everyone Juicing!

I've got most of my family juicing, at BBQs or dinners I regularly make fresh lemonade! "Loop d' Loop" has turned into a common request in my household, especially when my sister visits and fancies a health kick.

I've completed my exams for a diploma in Holistic Nutrition and Dietetics and I want to complete Jason's Juice Therapy Course and Academy next. Juicing really has changed my life and I would really like to inspire others to make similar changes as the rewards are amazing. You cannot put a price on your health. For me juicing really is the best health insurance you can buy!

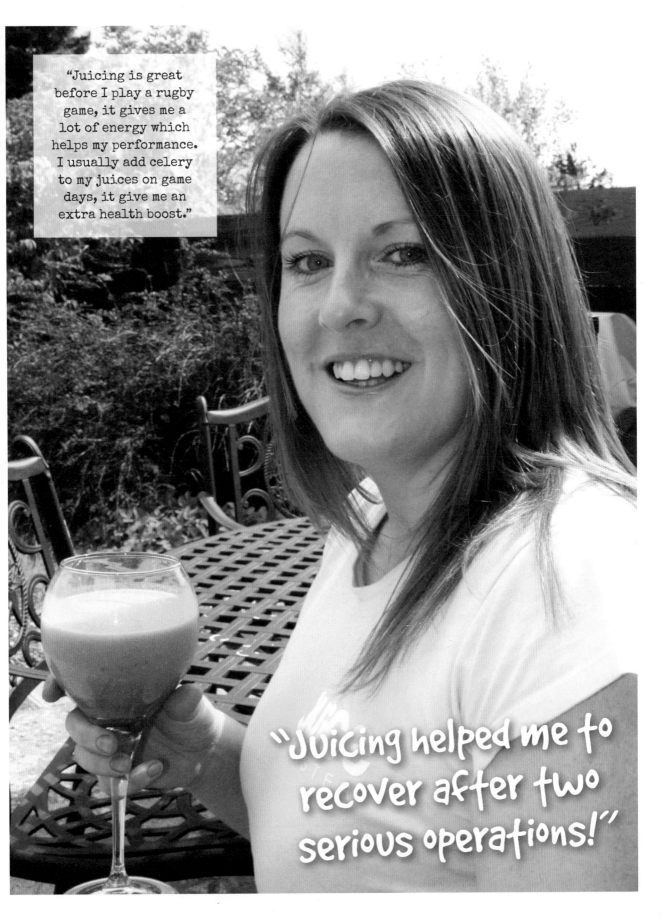

"Juicing is great before I play a rugby game, it gives me a lot of energy which helps my performance. I usually add celery to my juices on game days, it give me an extra health boost."

"Juicing helped me to recover after two serious operations!"

Dr Leigh Erin Connealy
Perfectly Healthy Mega Greens

I always use organic produce

2 cups spinach
2 limes – peeled
½ avocado
1 grapefruit
½ medium cucumber
1 Tbsp green super food powder optional
1-2 Tsp natural sweetener optional
1 Tbsp Vanilla Protein Powder optional
Handful of ice

Why not use JM Hemp Protein Powder

Juice the grapefruit, limes and spinach and blend together with the avocado, ice and other optional ingredients to taste. By adding the green super food powder it gives the smoothie a real veggie boost.

Raw honey, Stevia, or add an apple to the juice

As an MD, I treat everything from the common cold to cancer. I recommend juicing protocols to each and every patient, as part of a healthy lifestyle. I do this because I realized that conventional medicine had very limited returns and did not always improve the health of my patients.

I realized that conventional medicine had very limited returns and did not always improve health.

As an MD... I recommend juicing protocols to each and every patient.

At my clinic, we integrate detox protocols into each patient's plan. The Juice Master detox protocols – like those described in Jason Vale's book, 7lbs in 7 Days – are great and easy to do. A patient with high blood pressure or fatty liver, for example, can get tremendous benefits from juicing. In fact, most patients who follow my juicing recommendations have successfully reversed their symptoms.

Many patients can change and turn around their health using the one-step-at-a-time method to get their health back on track. It is so satisfying for me to see a patient who walked into my clinic with so many challenges finally able to sleep like a baby again, think clearly, enjoy exercising, balance stress, and simply enjoy life as it comes!

I feel that we must treat the patient with the disease and not the disease of the patient.

One thing is for sure – I embrace a healthy lifestyle myself, so juicing is an integral part of life for my family and me.

You can find out more about Dr. Connealy and her clinic at www.perfectlyhealthy.com

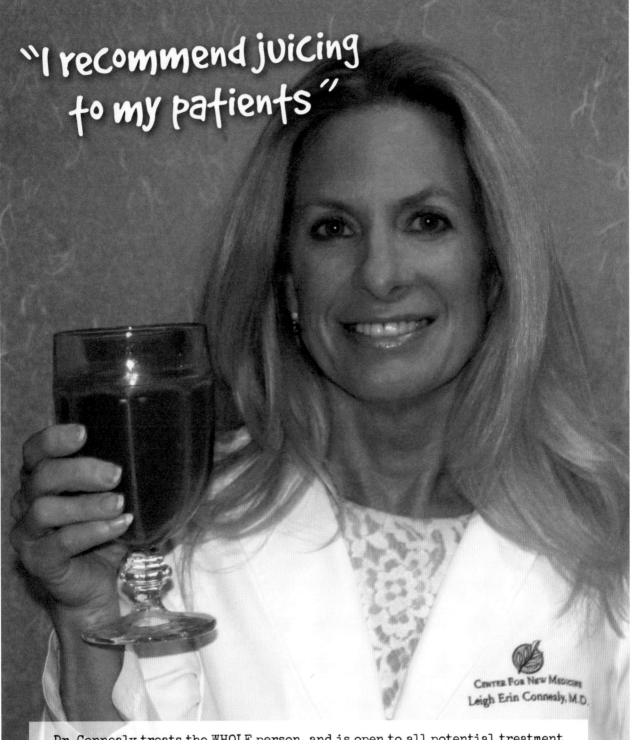

"I recommend juicing to my patients"

Dr. Connealy treats the WHOLE person, and is open to all potential treatment possibilities. She has over twenty years of experience in finding the 'root cause of an illness', and has taken numerous advanced courses, including homeopathic, nutritional and lifestyle approaches, while studying disease, chronic illness, and cancer treatments. She has a true passion to change her patients' lives, and give them their life back.

Kate Beswick's
Something For The Weekend

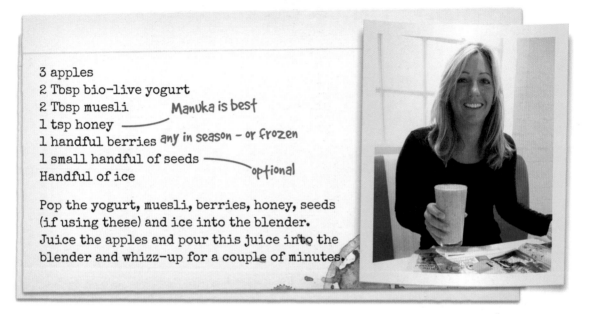

3 apples
2 Tbsp bio-live yogurt
2 Tbsp muesli
1 tsp honey — *Manuka is best*
1 handful berries *any in season – or frozen*
1 small handful of seeds
Handful of ice *optional*

Pop the yogurt, muesli, berries, honey, seeds
(if using these) and ice into the blender.
Juice the apples and pour this juice into the
blender and whizz-up for a couple of minutes.

OK so the reason I made it into the book is because I'm Jason's girlfriend (and work colleague)! Unlike most of the Juicy Community I don't have a radical juicing story to tell, but I do have a superb smoothie that I would love to share with you.

Juicing is Jason's hobby as well as his business, and over the years I have witnessed first hand how his mission to "juice the world" has grown from an idealistic dream to a very honest reality.

It's astounding to see the transformation in people – it's about taking control of your health

I feel so blessed to live and work with Jason and to be part of this juicy revolution. Every day we get numerous letters from people with extraordinary stories of how juicing has changed their lives. I spend several months a year working at our magical retreat in Turkey and it's astounding to see the transformation in people. Juicing is about far more than creating a drink, it's an opportunity to take control of your health.

I personally adore veggie juices and most days I combine cucumber, celery, lime, beetroot, ginger, spinach and apple. If I can't get a breakfast juice then my second choice is muesli or granola with berries, seeds and soya milk.

I love this particular smoothie because it's a combination of juice and muesli, it may sound odd, but I guarantee it tastes delicious. I love the texture and taste of muesli so I don't blend the smoothie for very long. If my smoothie were cooked veggies, then I would like them *al dente*, but you may prefer yours "well done" – so blend for as long as you like, it's your call.

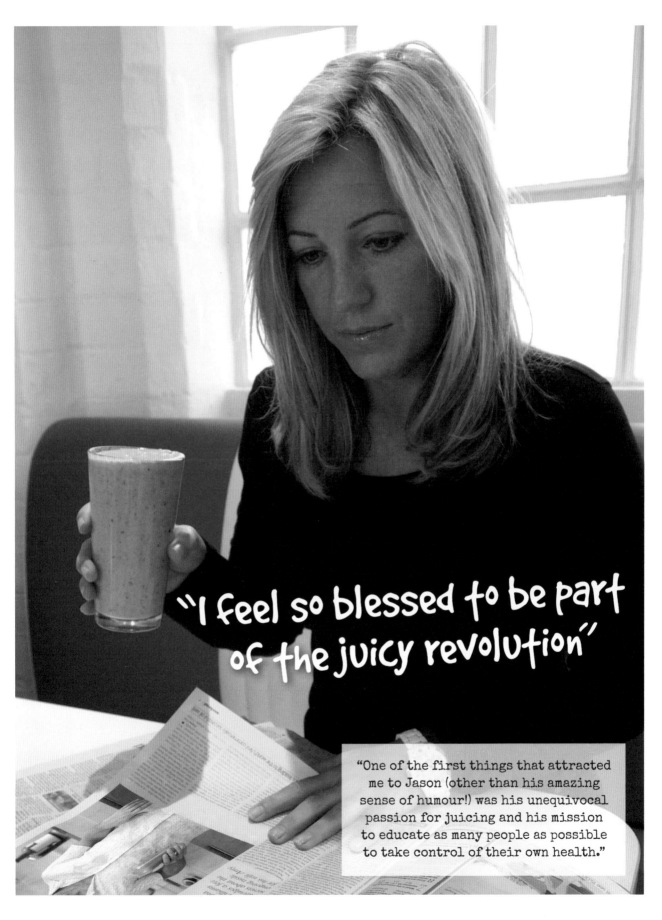

"I feel so blessed to be part of the juicy revolution"

"One of the first things that attracted me to Jason (other than his amazing sense of humour!) was his unequivocal passion for juicing and his mission to educate as many people as possible to take control of their own health."

Jason's Fave
Passion 4 Juice

come and share your passion for juice at Juicy oasis in Portugal

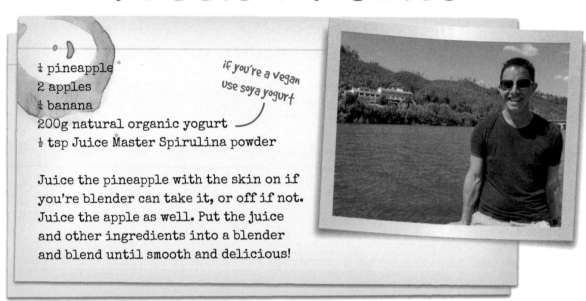

¼ pineapple
2 apples
¼ banana
200g natural organic yogurt — *if you're a vegan use soya yogurt*
½ tsp Juice Master Spirulina powder

Juice the pineapple with the skin on if you're blender can take it, or off if not. Juice the apple as well. Put the juice and other ingredients into a blender and blend until smooth and delicious!

My team suggested I should be in the Community Juice section and add my favourite recipe. The challenge with this is that it's rather like trying to pick your favourite film; it all depends on the category. For example I **love** *Finding Nemo*. It has to be one of, if not the finest animated film ever made (followed closely by *The Incredibles* and *Bolt*) – but would it win my "Best Ever" film award? Nope! I have no idea what film would in fact win. *Good Will Hunting? Lost In Translation? Finding Neverland?* The list goes on and I love each for their own reasons.

It's Impossible To Pick My "Favourite" Juice or Smoothie

It's the same with juices and smoothies, it's almost impossible to choose a definitive number one. However, if I "HAD" to choose then my absolute number one in the veggie world has to be the "Turbo Charge Smoothie" which is in my book *Turbo Charge Your Life In 14 Days* and also in *7lbs in 7 Days Super Juice Diet.*

Share In My Passion 4 Juice

But for this book, I've chosen my favourite fruit smoothie "Passion 4 Juice" because it isn't a hard-core health juice, it just tastes amazing! It's served on the morning of day three of the 7 day programme and trust me, after two full days on veggie based juices, this little baby always tastes better than pumpkin pie!

A Little Dash of Spirulina!

What I also love is that it has a little Spirulina. This turns it a lovely shade of green, adds heaps of veggie goodness, yet at the same time it still tastes like a dessert. Ticks every box and has made it in as my fave fruit-based smoothie - Enjoy!

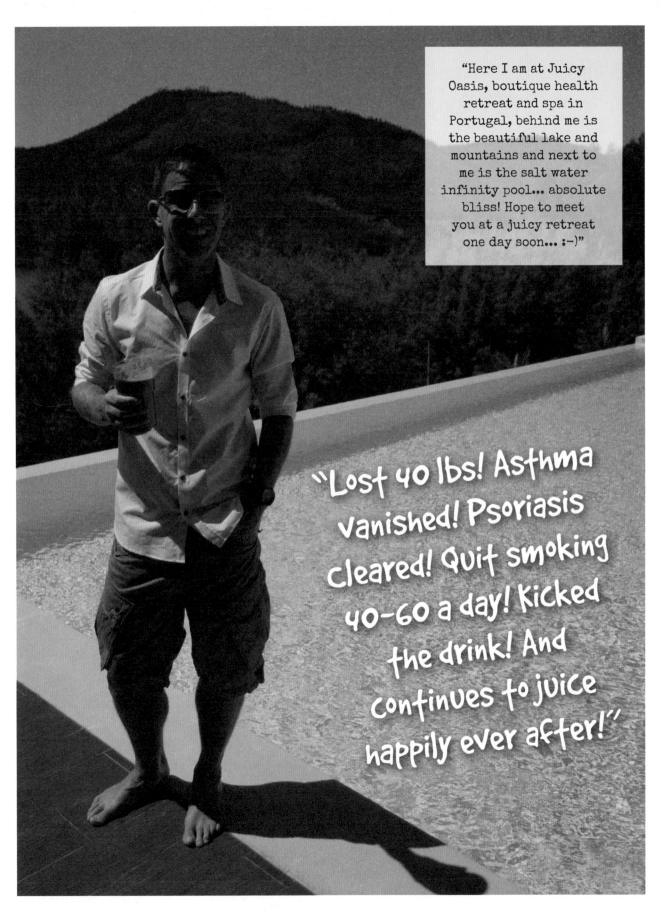

"Here I am at Juicy Oasis, boutique health retreat and spa in Portugal, behind me is the beautiful lake and mountains and next to me is the salt water infinity pool... absolute bliss! Hope to meet you at a juicy retreat one day soon... :-)"

"Lost 40 lbs! Asthma vanished! Psoriasis cleared! Quit smoking 40-60 a day! Kicked the drink! And continues to juice happily ever after!"

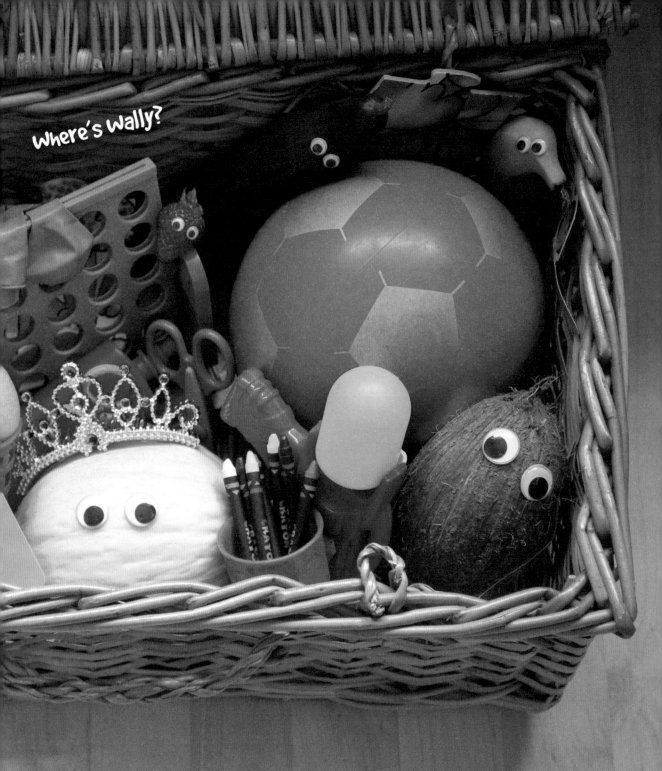

Where's Wally?

Thank You To All The Little
Juicers Who Contributed

Kidz Corner

"If You Can't Get Them To Eat It... Get Them To Drink It!"

One thing I believe the vast majority of people agree with is children require the finest nutrition available. The challenge, as I am sure you are aware, is that children aren't always as open to having raw broccoli as perhaps we would like. It appears they take a great deal more notice of what "Mr Ronald Mc D." and "Mr Ben & Jerry" have to say. Plus, and I feel it's fair to say, a Ben & Jerry's ice cream is just ever so slightly more appealing to the average kid than a raw carrot!

This Is Where Juicing And Smoothie Making Really Comes Into Its Own

Not only can you "disguise" certain raw veggies into a juice that looks and tastes like berries, but juicing brings a form of theatre to the breakfast table; a kind of experience which pouring milk onto cereal just doesn't!

Children love becoming the creators of their own concoctions and I have found over the years, that if they make it, no matter what the ingredients, they will always say they love it and they will always drink it. You may wish, however, to suggest certain ingredients as you go, as you will *also* be expected to drink whatever they make *and you will have to finish it all!*

In this section you will find a few wonderful concoctions from some of the children who are part of our juicy community. Some I know personally and others are part of what I call our "extended juicy family". We have tasted every juice and smoothie at Juicy HQ and we can safely say, they are all pretty special. I cannot encourage you enough to get the kids involved. The younger they are, the more amazed they seem as they watch a hard vegetable like a carrot, turn into juice before their eyes!

It's Possible To Get Your Little Ones To Drink Vegetable Juice

If you cannot encourage your little one to juice anything other than an apple and just the sight of raw broccoli going into the juice is enough to make them run a mile, here's a little trick. Firstly sweeten the juice with apple or pineapple. Always add raw beetroot (and broccoli, celery, cucumber, spinach, etc.) away from their little eyes. The juice is then deep red and looks like a berry juice. Bring the juice out and ask "Do you like berries?" to which they will of course reply "Yes!" Hand them the juice and say, "well if you love berries you will love this!"

Now please notice I have not lied, I have simply used misdirection. The question about berries was simply a random question. Even if you do "lie" to your child for the greater good every now and then, I really don't see any harm – especially as they will 100% lie to you at some stage when they are older! I realise this stops them getting involved but if they really won't make a veggie juice this is the way to get it into them. You can still encourage them to make fruit juices and now and then

Alfie's
Smashing Strawberry

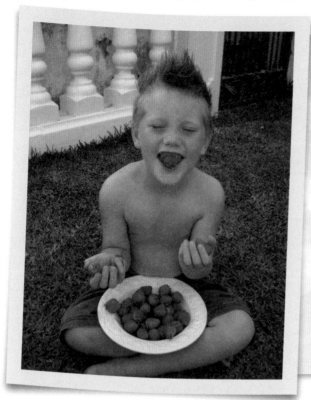

2 golden delicious apples
1 banana
1 handful strawberries

Juice the apples, put the juice in a blender and add the banana and strawberries (try not to eat all the strawberries before you put them in).

Blend it all up!

"My favourite fruit is strawberries. I love to watch them turn creamy in the blender with the banana. My Smashing Strawberry is the bestest tasting drink in the whole wide world. I really love it and it's healthy"

Little Strawberry Facts

Strawberries are the only fruit with the seeds on the outside! Fresh strawberries, like the ones in this juice are incredibly rich in vitamin C with is a powerful antioxidants.

Here's Alfie, brother of the lovely Molly (across the page there) and one of the cutest kids you'll ever come across. He tweaks the nose of terror and drops ice cubes down the pants of fear (as Black Adder would say). What I mean is: he has no fear and my prediction is he will end up as a sportsman of some kind.

Alfie has recently got into football and his very own smoothie is loaded with potassium and sodium, which is great because these are two vital minerals lost when doing exercise like footie.

A great tasting juice by a really cool young man!

Molly's
Sunrise Special

2 apples
¼ lime
½ inch of ginger
4 carrots
1 inch cucumber
¼ pineapple

Juice it all up with a
juicer and enjoy my
delicious sunshine juice!!

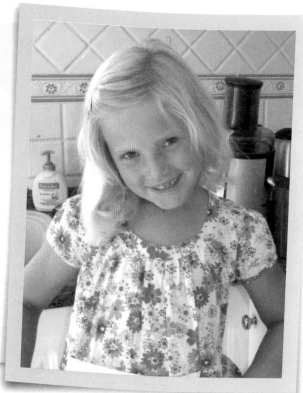

Here is my beautiful little niece Molly. She got into juicing when she was just two years old. Molly would come next door to my partner Kate's gorgeous converted barn in Cornwall, stand on the work surface and push through some fruit and veggies (supervised of course!). Ever since then she has loved making her own juicy concoctions and is a big juicing fan.

Molly is currently living in Spain, enjoying the sunshine and of course her "Sunrise Special" juice. Not only does it taste creamy and delicious, it's packed with specific nutrients required to help a growing mind and body...

Thank you little Molly for sharing your favourite juice with everyone.

"It's so creamy,
it's so juicy,
lick your lips,
for Jason's Juicy!"

Look What's In Molly's Juice

Vitamins: A, B, B1, B2, B3, B6, C, E, K. A great combination of essential vitamins, you're sure to feel full of sunshine after one of these!

Poppy's
Poppy Power

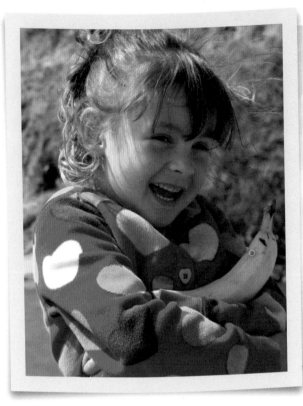

1 handful strawberries
1 handful blackberries
1 handful raspberries
1 banana
1 slice melon
1 handful ice

First we go to the shop and get the ingredients. Next you put it all in a blender and turn it into a smoothie. Oh... remember to pour it into a glass and add a big bendy-straw.

"I like Jason because he likes juicing.
I like Jason because he is healthy.
I love Juicy Kate because she is funny.
I like juicing because I can drink my veg".

This is little Poppy. She is one of the most adorable kidz I know. Always happy, always smiling and a joy to be around. I took this picture of her when I was hanging out in Cornwall writing this book. I asked if she would share a gorgeous recipe for us all and here it is. I am sure little Pops only drinks this because it taste gorgeous, but it's worth knowing that this is one of the most antioxidant-rich smoothies in the book. It is especially rich in B vitamins, of which we require 13 for human nutrition. Vitamin B6 is one of the most frequently deficient vitamins and this smoothie is rich in this vitamin. This vitamin alone helps to produce antibodies for the immune system, is active in the metabolism of amino acids, and releases glucose from the liver.

Thank you Pops for an amazing tasting and incredibly good for you smoothie.

"I am Poppy and I am 6, I like juicing because it is fun and making smoothies with Mummy because they are yummy."

Dylan's
Juicylicious Ogre

2 apples
¼ pineapple
½ parsnip
1 handful of parsley
1 handful of spinach
1 inch ginger
¼ lemon
1 handful crushed ice

Juice all the ingredients, pour over crushed ice and enjoy! Remember, it might be an ogre juice but you don't have to make a mess like one.

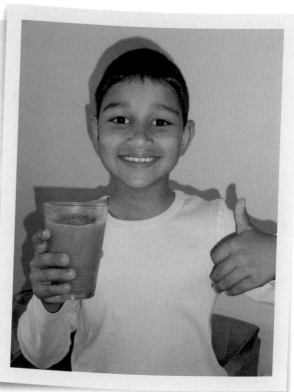

Nina Chauhan has been with my company pretty much from the beginning. Every now and then I would see her son Dylan popping his head in the office. "A bundle of pure energy" is perhaps the only way to describe him. This picture of him smiling from ear to ear pretty much sums him up: one happy juicer!

Dylan has kindly donated one of his favourite recipes to the juicy cause, which he describes as "juicylicious".

It's an unusual set of ingredients – parsley and raw parsnip may not be the first choice of most 6 year olds, but mixed with apple and pineapple and they add to the overall gorgeous taste and creaminess. Thanks Dylan – "you da man"!

"My juice is tangy, my juice is sweet,
It's even got veg I don't usually eat!
Drink it yourself, you'll love it as well,
It's a yummy creation,
taste, texture and smell!"

Parsnips in a juice?

Well it is an ogre juice, and if I was an ogre I would definitely eat (or juice) them as they're full of Vitamins C, B3 and E along with essential carbohydrates and dietary fibre.

Scout's
Smarty Tarty

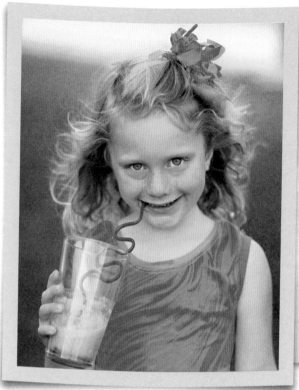

2 apples
1 small slice pineapple
½ small lemon (peeled)
½ small lime (peeled)
2 inch cucumber
1 inch courgette
1 inch broccoli stem
handful spinach
handful ice

Juice all the ingredients,
pour over ice cubes into
a shaker bottle and shake
it up so it's all blended
and nice and cool.

"Scout loves pouring her juice into a shaker bottle and sometimes even doing a little dance while shaking it" – Heidi (mum)

My name is Heidi and I have a four year-old, very picky, daughter called Scout. Getting her to eat vegetables is an on-going struggle, but she always happily drinks juice.

When I was doing the Juice Master 7 and 3 day plans, she loved trying the juices. Some days, she'd ask me to make an entire new one for her! She loves the colours and the vibrant flavours. I love that she's having vegetables and enjoying them!

Like me, she loves tart and acidic tastes so I developed a recipe for her with the tartness she loves and some easily disguisable veggies for me :). That's why we decided to call it 'Smarty Tarty."

I usually pour the well-blended juice into a pretty cup and serve with her favourite straw.

Courgettes – or as they're known in other parts of the world Zucchini – are available all year round but are at their best in the late spring or early summer seasons.

Don't confuse a courgette for a marrow, they don't taste as good.

Max's
Monster Max

2 apples
½ banana
¼ pineapple
1 small raw beetroot
1 tablespoon natural yogurt
½ avocado

Juice the apples and pineapple. Add the juice to the blender with the banana, yogurt, avocado and ice. Blend it all up! Pour into a tall glass until half full. Juice the beetroot then slowly add it to the middle of the juice, then top up with more of the first juice.

"Juice, then blend and at the end dribble in the beetroot juice. 'Wow' is Max's favourite word for this monster of a juice" – John (dad).

Hi I'm dad John and this is my son Max, he's 4, he's great and he loves his juice.

After trying loads of different things to get Max to have his 5-a-day, we found the best way was to juice the fruit and veg; and then name the juice – the funkier, more colourful and wackier the better! We find this the easiest way for Max to get the healthy foods he needs (we slip in as many greens as possible).

Max loves inventing and making juices himself. He really enjoys seeing the blender whizz-up the ingredients and watching the colours change as he feeds raw beetroot into the juicer; and then minutes later drinking it! We thought this would never happen, but Max proved us wrong!

Max had eczema from an early age and a dislike for all foods, we had a challenge to get him eating anything let alone the healthier stuff. But allowing Max to make his own juices and sticking everything from raw broccoli, beetroot, carrots, apples, avocado and bananas through a juicer or blender really has got him excited about tasting and experimenting with his food. Maybe he'll even be doing his own recipe book soon!

Yasmine's
Magical Smoothie

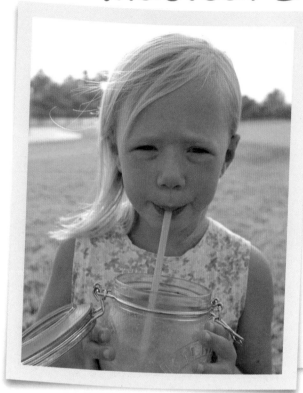

2 apples
½ medium pineapple
1 handful strawberries
2 heaped Tbsp bio-live yogurt
1 handful ice

Juice the apples and pineapple, blend together with the strawberries, bio-live yogurt and ice. Serve in your favourite glass and slurp it up through a straw.

Yummy, yummy, strawberries,
Yummy in my tummy,
I love my magic smoothie,
Made freshly by my mummy!

Hi I'm Claire and I am Yasmine's Mummy. This smoothie contains one of Yasmine's favourite fruits – strawberries! She takes a freshly made smoothie to school every day here in Dubai, which is where she lives with me, her Daddy and little brother Ethan. Yasmine became interested in juices and smoothies when I started juicing just over a year ago as just one of the ways I started fighting my stage four breast cancer. She started helping me juice and became the family's official taste tester – nudging her Daddy out of the running (who is in fact a Chef!).

She developed a taste for the veggie juices as well as the fruit juices and smoothies. She particularly liked the green ones and the beetroot ones – much to my surprise! She likes to experiment with new flavours and often invites her little friends round to try out her creations, making them guess the ingredients, which this is always good fun!

I recently went to Jason's new Juicy Oasis in Portugal and next year Yasmine has decided she wants to go too! Yasmine's favourite phrase after making this smoothie is "this is the bestest day ever!". Well, she is only 5!

Aston's
The Joker

3 pears
1 small raw beetroot
ice

Simply juice the lot
and pour over ice.

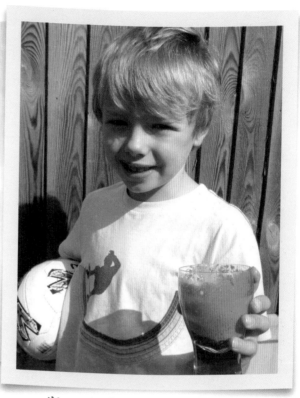

This is Aston, he's 7 years old and loves juicing, with a little help from me – his mother Skye. The Joker is his favourite breakfast juice, the combination of ingredients, especially the beetroot (a great blood builder) helps Aston to start his day in the best possible way.

Aston says "I like juicing because it's healthy and when I grow up I want to be healthy and strong". Aston is very sporty and a huge football fan of Chelsea. He plays for his local team, Brentwood Athletic FC and trains with them once a week, plus at school, in the garden and even indoors! He will have a juice before training to give him "extra power" on the pitch!

"I made this juice up myself. I love the colour of it, I called it 'The Joker' because it gives me a big red Joker smile!"

I'm a personal trainer and a keen runner. I love sharing the benefits of raw juices with others. I've even been to Aston's school to do a juicing demo for his class, helping his classmates understand that there is another way to ingest some of the less popular vegetables, which are easily hidden in a delicious juice!

"Juicing is so cool!"

Emily's
Tiger Smoothie

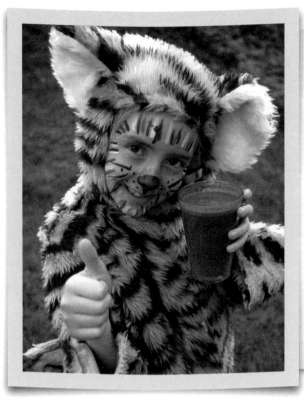

1 banana (ripe)
2 cups oat milk
1 tsp raw cacao powder
2 tsp organic runny-honey

It's a smoothie so no juicing is needed - just a blender! Put all the ingredients into the blender and blend it up 'til lovely and smooth.

*"Watch out there's a tiger about,
It wants to swipe your smoothie,
It likes the creamy, healthy, taste,
It thinks your smoothie's groovy!"*

Hi I'm Charlie and this is my daughter Emily. She's a very lovely, energetic little girl who loves jumping about and playing very active games. She's a huge fan of nature and loves tigers and big cats.

Considering how much energy Emily has you may be surprised to hear that she doesn't like fruit or veg. From the beginning, when she was weaned from breast milk, she didn't take to them and she's never really grown out of it.

And we've tried everything to get her to eat her 5 a day: we've smushed it up; disguised it; given it funny names; hidden it in soups; let her play with it; let her prepare it; set a good example ourselves; encouraged her; educated her... but nothing seems to make her actually want to eat her greens or any other colour for that matter.

Then we started to juice and we were surprised to find that she would (sometimes) have one – and like it! Hallelujah!! She's not very adventurous but there are a couple of juices and smoothies she will now have on a regular basis and as a mother I feel I can breathe a sigh of relief.

Tiger Smoothie is her favourite, it takes something naughty and turns it into something (a tiny bit) more nutritious.

Ethan's
Super Summer Sherbert

2 royal gala apples
¼ pineapple (no skin)
½ lemon

Juice everything and pour into a nice tall glass. No! Don't juice "everything", that would be silly – just the ingredients need juicing!

"I love making up my own juices and I like vegetables more in juice form than eating them. Shhhhhh! don't tell my mum but I've even had avocado in a juice before!"

Hi I'm Ethan's dad, Alex. I introduced juicing to the family when Ethan was 7, after I had a bout of IBS, myself. It's definitely become a way of life in our household, and now Ethan's 11 he's pretty independent about making his own juices. He loves to prep the fruit and veg, make the juice and share it out... although he's still not too enthusiastic about cleaning up afterwards!

Super Summer Sherbet is Ethan's invention for the summer. It has a really nice frothy head and tastes wonderfully sherberty, perfect for hot summer days. He did try adding raspberries to the juice (he likes eating them); it made it go a wonderful pink lemonade colour and we all loved

it – apart from Ethan! It turns out he didn't like raspberries in the juice. Still, he did say "I guess it's good to try new things out". Experimenting with juice recipes has definitely made him braver about trying other healthy foods. He rarely has cooked vegetables, preferring raw carrots, apples, celery and cucumber with his main meal.

"I hope you like my juice as much as I do!" – Ethan

Emily's
Excellent Energiser

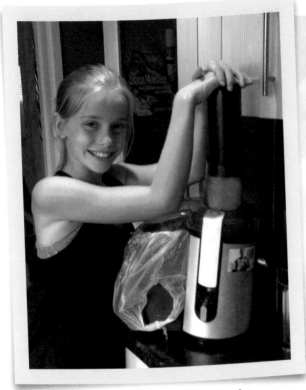

1 orange (peeled)
¼ pineapple
½ mango (ripe and peeled)
1 Tbsp natural yogurt
1 Tsp honey

Juice the pineapple
and orange and blend
up with the mango,
yogurt and honey until
beautifully smooth.

*"Emily is an athlete in the making...
she wants to be an olympic
star." - Victoria (mum)*

This is Emily and she's an athlete in the making. She loves sport and has so much energy. Emily raves about juicing because not only does it taste yummy, she knows it's giving her all the nutrient's she needs to help her hopefully become the next Olympic star.

Her mum Victoria said, "It is so easy for kids these days to pick up unhealthy food. Juicing has really changed how our family see food and we all fight over the juicer in the morning! Emily is so passionate about athletics and runs everywhere, so we realise

how important it is to give her all the fruits and vegetables to keep her energy high."

The ancient Romans and Greeks referred to honey as "food fit for the Gods" and as an olympian in the making it's understandable that honey play a part.

The bees that produce the honey are athletes in themselves visiting a staggering 50-100 flowers per nectar gathering trip!

Adam, Toby & Sam's
Brother Nature

3 apples
3 pears
1 Tbsp milled flax seeds
1 mango
4 Tbsp bio-live yogurt
ice

Juice the apples and pears.
Put the flax seeds, mango,
yogurt and ice into the
blender. Blend until smooth.

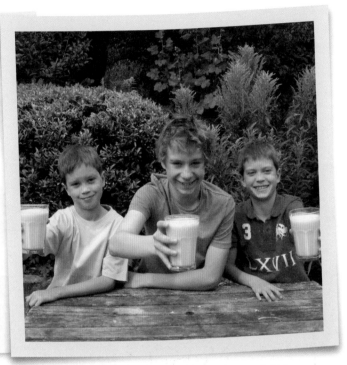

Adam just got into Eton and this
super brain smoothie is just
what he needs for his studies.

This is Adam, (in the middle aged 14) sandwiched by his brothers – the terrible twins (Toby and Sam both aged 10 – well they are twins so unsure the explanation of both being the same age was necessary).

The twins do tend to pick on Adam a bit, so if you are reading this – stop it! :-) Watch out for Toby and Sam Duffen: you just may see them playing for your favourite football club in the future! One's a left-footer, one's a right – it appears the new Neville Brother's are on their way! I think also being son's of Paul Duffen, who once helped Hull FC to reach the Premiership, might help too.

As for Adam, well he's just been accepted into Eton, which is no mean feat, and his choice of smoothie is certainly one which will help to feed his brain. Milled flax seed breaks down Omega-3 essential oils for your body to absorb. Unlike whole flax seed (which cannot be digested) there are some who claim it's one of the most powerful plant foods on the planet and there's some evidence that it can help reduce your risk of heart disease, cancer, stroke, and diabetes. It is also said to help brain development. However, with Adam already in Eton I'm unsure what further help he needs. :-)

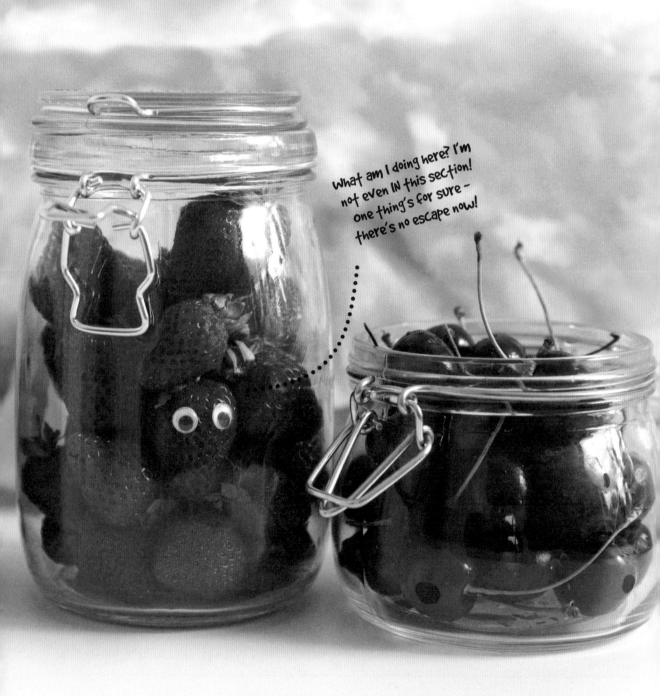

The Candy Store

When I was growing up I was, let's say, a little partial to anything which tasted sweet and creamy. This contributed largely to me looking like a little fat pigeon back in those days! All these years later and, although now fond of the green and healthy, I am still human and love a little sweet treat.

The Following Recipes Are Deliciously Sweet & Creamy, & Will Make You Feel Naughty!

However, although these recipes taste too good to be healthy – they still are. Okay, they might not be quite in the same league as "The Ultimate Veggie Breakfast" (p. 99), but they're all still loaded with nutrients. So although it may feel like you're doing something really bad, your body will still love you for it… to some degree ;-)

A Little Warning…

The smoothies in The Candy Store are effectively a "meal in a glass" and ideally shouldn't be consumed after a meal, but rather as a meal in themselves!

"THEY TASTE TOO GOOD TO BE GOOD FOR YOU"

"LIKE DROPLETS OF HEAVEN ON YOUR TONGUE"

"DELICIOUS & NUTRITIOUS"

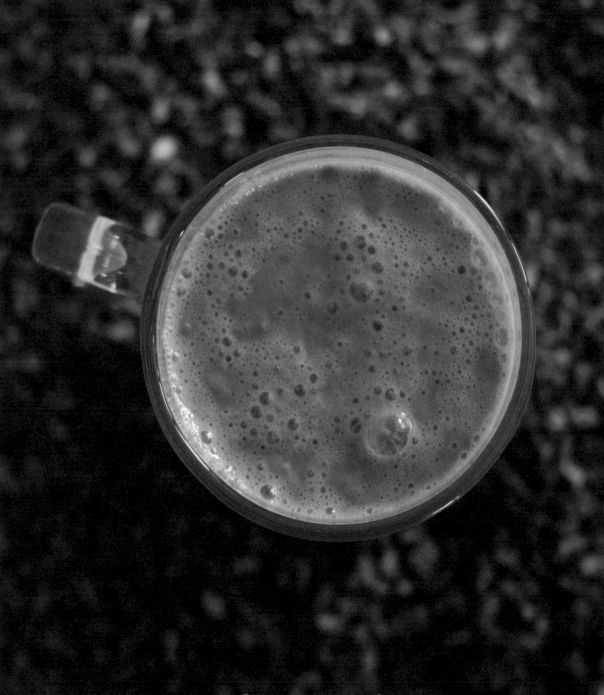

Cocoa-tastic!

Did you know that a cup of cocoa has almost three
times the antioxidants of a cup of green tea?!

Tahini Choco Beaney

In the style of Chitty Chitty Bang Bang this smoothie is "Truly Scrumptious" and should satisfy the cravings of even the biggest choco-head! Dense raw cocoa extract blended with deliciously nutty tahini, creamy banana, a swirl of honey and a splash of almond milk.

Fairtrade Raw Cocoa Powder
1 tablespoon

Tahini
1 tablespoon

Manuka Honey
2 teaspoons

Banana
½ (ripe & peeled)

Almond Milk
250ml

Ice Cubes
1 small handful

Tahini Bo-Beaney

This is "Truly Simple" to make! Just add all the ingredients to the blender and whizz-up until "Smoothly Scrumptious".

Best Served... when you feel like indulging in something chocolatey and sweet and devilishly delicious.

Can I Remotely Justify This?

Absolutely you can! Tahini is a great source of calcium, magnesium, iron, phosphorus, zinc, vitamins B1, B2, B3, B5 and pangamic acid.

B vitamins play an essential part in the running of the body. They promote healthy cell growth and division, including red blood cells, which helps prevent anaemia.

Cocoa is the powder of the raw cacao bean and is as far away (on a health front) from mass produced, sugar loaded commercial chocolate as Mary Poppins is from Lord Voldemort. It is renowned for its high anti-oxidant levels and is believed to enhance mood, lower blood pressure and reduce the risk of heart disease and strokes.

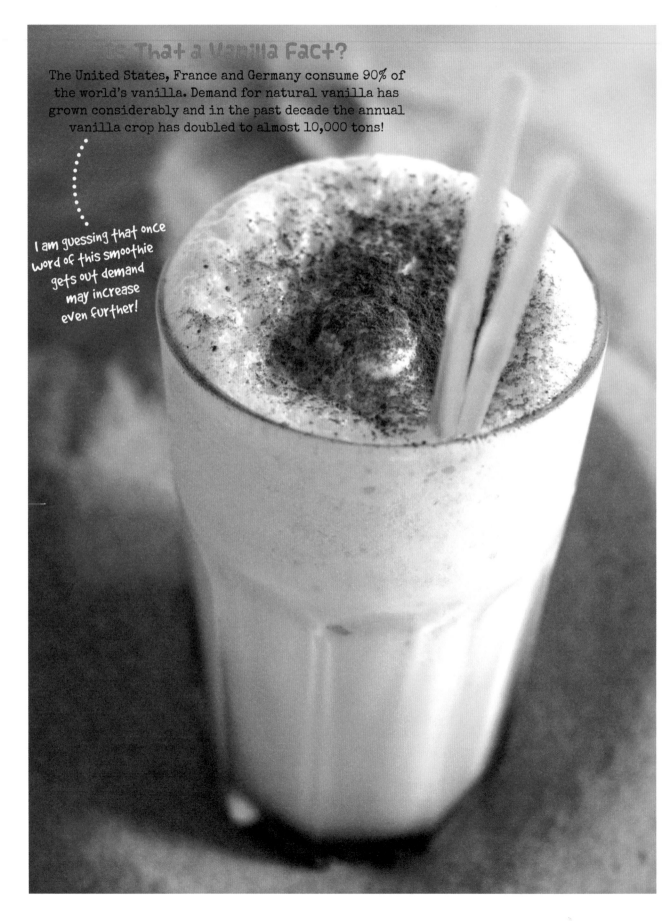

Is That a Vanilla Fact?

The United States, France and Germany consume 90% of the world's vanilla. Demand for natural vanilla has grown considerably and in the past decade the annual vanilla crop has doubled to almost 10,000 tons!

I am guessing that once word of this smoothie gets out demand may increase even further!

Vanilla Ice Cream Smoothie

I've always **loved** vanilla ice cream ever since it first danced on my tongue. Unfortunately, the problem with ice cream is that it's loaded with sugar. So I have come up with a (relatively) healthy alternative.

Hope you and the little ones **love it as much as I do**!

Pineapple
½

Golden Delicious Apple
1

Vanilla Pod
seeds from 1

Bio-Live Yogurt
4 large tablespoons

Manuka (Active) Honey
1 heaped teaspoon

Ice Cubes
1 small handful

Fairtrade Raw Cocoa Powder
light dusting (optional)

Sweet Instructions

Juice the pineapple (no need to peel if you have a good juicer – although you get a smoother juice if you peel it) and the apple.

Slice the vanilla pod and scrape the seeds directly into the blender. Add the fresh juice, yogurt, honey and ice, and blend until creamy and mind-blowingly delicious.

Best Served... over a large scoop of crushed ice – we want it to be icy and creamy... as in Ice Cream!

Too Tasty To Be Healthy?

It's true that this tastes too good to be healthy, but look what's in it: vitamins A, B1, B2, B3, B6, Folic Acid, C, E, and K; minerals including potassium, iron, sodium, calcium, zinc, magnesium, phosphorous, selenium, copper and manganese. It also contains digestive enzymes, natural sugars, amino acids, essential fatty acids, and many other amazing things that I'm sure science has yet to uncover!

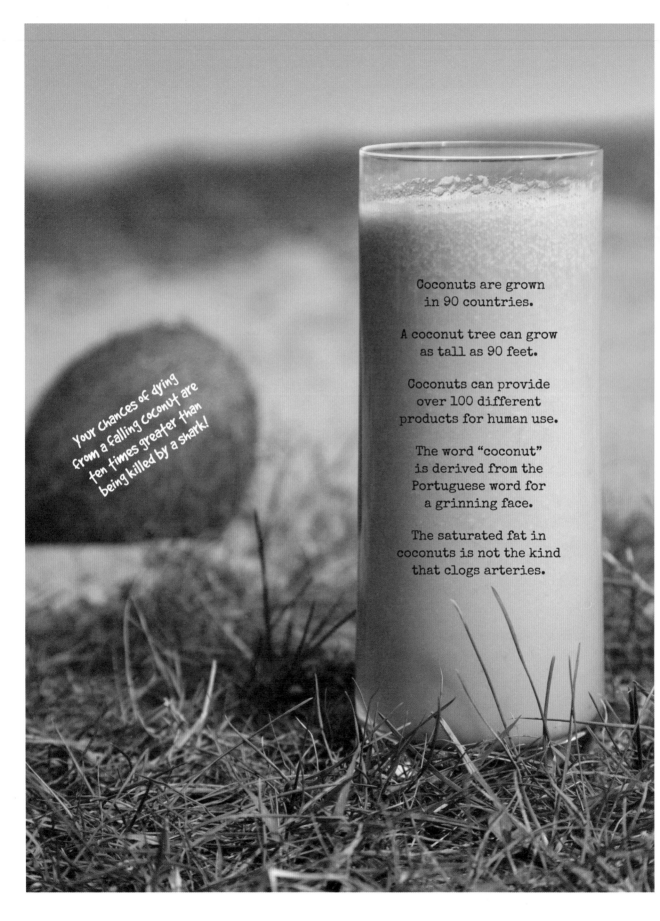

Your chances of dying from a falling coconut are ten times greater than being killed by a shark!

Coconuts are grown in 90 countries.

A coconut tree can grow as tall as 90 feet.

Coconuts can provide over 100 different products for human use.

The word "coconut" is derived from the Portuguese word for a grinning face.

The saturated fat in coconuts is not the kind that clogs arteries.

Coconut Heaven

Sensual, divine, creamy, rich and incredibly indulgent, this is not just a smoothie this is a "Juice Master **Angels Dancing On Your Taste Buds**" smoothie, (yes, I know it's taken from a very old advert – but hey, come on!)

Golden Delicious Apples
2

Unwaxed Lime
1

Coconut Milk
150 ml

Banana
½ (ripe & peeled)

Manuka (Active) Honey
1 teaspoon

Ice Cubes
1 small handful

What Are You Waiting For?

Juice the apples and lime (no need to peel).

Pour the fresh juice into the blender. Add all the other ingredients to the blender and blend 'til smooth.

Best Served... on special heavenly occasions. Compared to a green vegetable smoothie, it wouldn't win any awards in the "Healthiest Smoothie of the Year" competition, so make this smoothie and enjoy it for all its fabulousness, but let's just keep it for *special* and not for everyday use!

This Coco-Can't Be Good For Me?

Coconut milk does contain saturated fat, but so does mothers milk, and both have many nourishing health properties. So please dump your preconceived fear of saturated fat – it's not all bad!

And honey is a wonderful alternative to white refined sugar and provides a fabulous boost of natural energy.

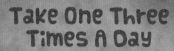

Take One Three Times A Day

In the past, blueberries were used for medicinal purposes (along with their leaves and roots) for treating coughs.

In recent times it has been discovered that blueberries (and other berries) may actually help to alleviate the cognitive decline in Alzheimer's disease.

Vanilla, Blueberry & Almond Indulgence

Blueberries tumbling and splashing into unadulterated creamy almond milk, combined with vanilla beans straight from the pod and topped off with thick creamy bio-live yogurt – *Indulgent? You bet!*

Vanilla Pod
seeds from 1

Fresh Blueberries
1 large handful

Almond Milk
250 ml

Bio-Live Yogurt
2 tablespoons

Ice Cubes
1 small handful

Instructions

Slice the vanilla pod and scrape the seeds directly into the blender. Add the blueberries, almond milk, yogurt and ice, and mix it up until smooth and creamy.

Best Served... when you are feeling rather pleased with yourself for finishing that piece of work on time; or getting that promotion; or finally plucking up the courage to ask that cute guy/girl out on a date. Sit back, savour this divine smoothie and reflect on your glorious achievement.

Why Almond Milk?

Almond milk is a combination of almonds and water, it is dairy free, cholesterol free, lactose free and contains high levels of protein, calcium, magnesium, potassium, manganese, copper, vitamin E and selenium. So although this smoothie tastes very indulgent, one of the side effects is its actually phenomenally nutrient rich. Happy, happy days!

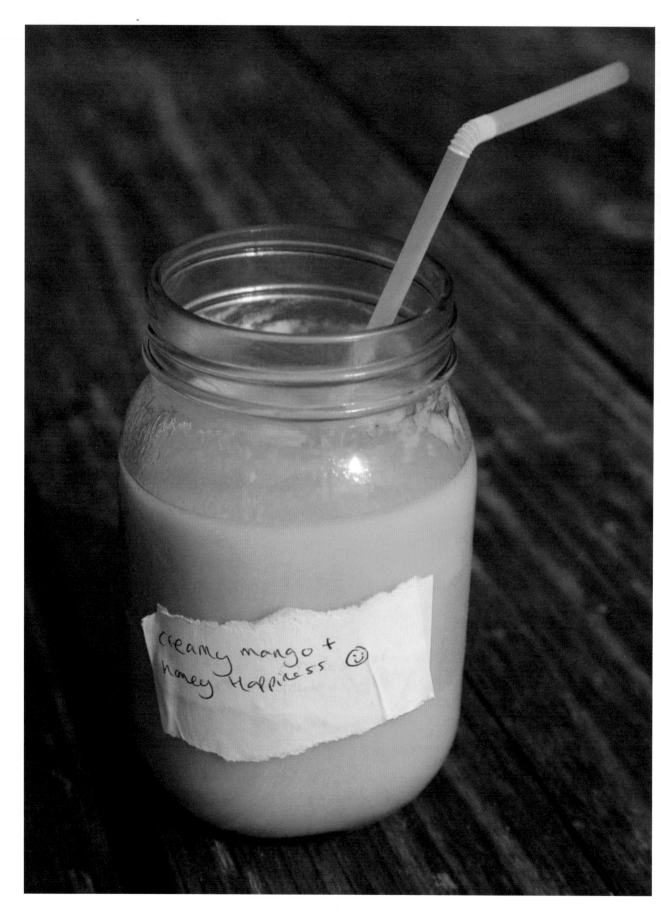

Creamy Mango & Honey Happiness

Sweet exotic pineapple juice blended with tropical mango, thick creamy yogurt and finished off with a generous dollop of Manuka active honey.

Pineapple
¾

Mango
½ (ripe, peeled & pitted)

Bio-Live Yogurt
2 tablespoons

Manuka (Active) Honey
1 heaped teaspoon

Ice Cubes
1 small handful

Let's Get Happy :-)

Juice the pineapple (with the skin on if your juicer will take it – although you get a smoother juice if you peel it).

Pour the fresh juice into the blender. Carefully slice the mango just off-centre, avoiding the large pit inside, then scoop the flesh into the blender. Add the yogurt, honey and ice, and blend until smooth and creamy.

Best Served... when the world has been mean to you and you feel the need to indulge in some inner happiness. Who needs Häagen-Dazs when you have "Creamy Mango and Honey Happiness"?!

How This Will Make You Happy!

If you have been avoiding mangoes due to the bad press from diet clubs – it's time to think again. Yes, mangoes are higher in calories than other fruits, but it's not a fair judgement. Put into perspective, half a mango contains 68 calories compared to 240 calories for a Cadburys Caramel bar! Personally, I think counting calories is nonsense anyway; but if you are into it, then this should give you peace of mind.

So get the juicy mango peeled and start enjoying some natural sweetness without the guilt!

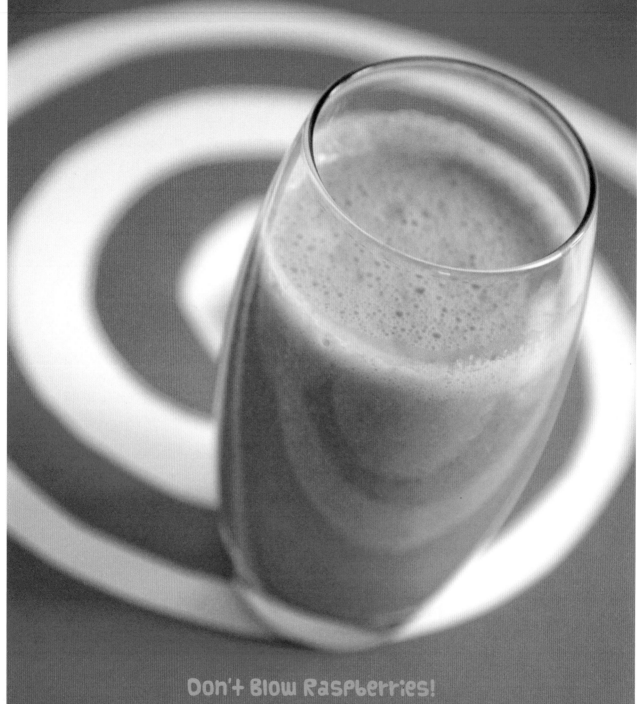

Don't Blow Raspberries!

If you can get hold of them "black raspberries" are not only
delicious, but also incredibly high in anthocyanins and have been
found by Ohio State University to be highly beneficial in treating
Barret's Oesophagus and preventing oesophageal cancer.

Raspberry Ripple

Delicate, soft, velvety raspberries blended with creamy fresh bio-live yogurt and delicious smooth pineapple juice. Sometimes your taste buds get sent on **an indescribable journey** – enjoy the trip!

Pineapple
⅔

Fresh Raspberries
1 large handful

Bio-Live Yogurt
2 tablespoons

Ice Cubes
1 small handful

A Ripple Of Deliciousness

Juice the pineapple (with the skin on if your juicer will take it – although you get a smoother juice if you peel it).

Pour the fresh juice into the blender. Then add the raspberries, yogurt, and ice, and blend until smooth.

Best Served... Any time day or night, especially when you're craving some raspberry ripple ice cream.

Reasons To Love Raspberries

According to research conducted in the Netherlands raspberries have 50% more antioxidants than strawberries and 10 times more than tomatoes and broccoli. Raspberries are an excellent source of manganese which promotes healthy bones and boosts metabolism.

They are also a very good source of vitamin C, which is vital for the immune system, and cell and tissue repair. The red pigment in raspberries is created by the anthocyanins which have anti-inflammatory properties that may also help reduce cardiovascular disease.

All this and they taste amazing too, so stop reading this and get yourself to the shop to stock up on your furry little friends!

Super Shots

The Small Shots With The Biggest Punch!

Good things come in small packages, as they say, and this is one of the cases where that saying holds some weight. This array of super juice shots pack an enormous amount of nutrition into a single shot! We live in a world where we believe a tiny medical synthetic pill or even vitamin pill, can do so much in terms of our health and yet we seem to think a little shot juice won't have much effect. Please do not underestimate the nutritional power of some of these super shots. The Garlic Shot for example, is perhaps the finest natural antibiotic you can take. It is also antiviral and antifungal and unlike drug antibiotics, it will not kill off our healthy bacteria. If you have any infections or fungal issues, get one of these down you every day until it clears. If the Garlic Shot is too much for you on the taste (and breath) front, try the Ginger Shot.

All these super shots are as powerful as the Garlic Shot in their own way. Some will require a powder (see "What'Supp?" on the following page). Don't go crazy with the shots; less is more when it comes to these mini powerhouses. I would highly recommend having a shot before your "main" juice of the day. Your juicer is going to need cleaning anyway, so have a shot then, for extra nutrition. I tend to opt for a ginger shot and berry shot, but the choice is yours clearly. I always have a wheatgrass shot too, but I have those delivered in ready-made frozen shots, which I simply take from the freezer, pop in water for 5 mins, open and drink (see wheatgrass page for more on this, p.254).

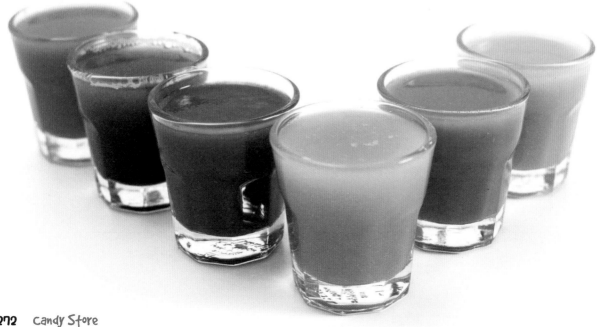

GINGER SHOT

½ large apple (or whole small)

5 cm chunk of ginger

Just juice, add to small shot glass and down in one!

This little shot was created by Kasper who owns the juice chain Joe and The Juice – thanks boys. It's a natural antiviral, antibiotic, antifungal, antihistamine, anti-inflammatory, antiseptic, increases blood flow, promotes sweating and relaxes peripheral blood vessels.

GARLIC SHOT

½ large apple (or whole small)

2 cloves garlic

Just juice, add to small shot glass and down in one!

Nature's finest antibiotic, antiviral and antifungal. If you have an infection or fungus in your nails, get one of these in you daily!

WHEATGRASS SHOT

The most famous "shot" in the world… after tequila! See the wheatgrass page for how to make your shot as there are several ways.

20 amino acids

11 x more calcium than cow's milk

5 x more iron than spinach

4 x the Vitamin B1 of whole-wheat flour

7 x the Vitamin C of oranges.

More protein than beef.

Excellent source of vitamin C, E, K, B complex.

Rich in calcium, cobalt, iron, magnesium, phosphorus, potassium, sodium, sulphur, and zinc. Rich in Chlorophyll.

SUPER BERRY SHOT

½ large apple (or whole small)

Heaped teaspoon of Ultimate Berry Powder

Juice the apple, pour into a protein shaker, add the powder and shake until dissolved. Pour into shot glass and knock back in one! (If you don't have a protein shaker, then just stir in).

Contains the highest antioxidant fruits in the world. Rich in amino acids, essential fats, vitamins, minerals and enzymes. Just the Acai Berries alone are described as, "the number one anti-ageing food" by Dr Nicholas Perricone. These berries are twice as potent as blueberries. Goji berries (also known as wolfberries) contain 500 x more vitamin C than oranges and more beta-carotene than carrots, as well being very rich in iron. That's just two of the berries!

SUPER GREEN SHOT

½ large apple (or whole small)

1 heaped teaspoon of Juice Master's Ultimate Super Food

Juice the apple, pour into a protein shaker, add the powder and shake until dissolved. Pour into a shot glass and knock back in one! (If you don't have a protein shaker, then just stir in.)

Contains the dried powders of all the green juices that matter: Whole Leaf Barley Grass, Whole Leaf Wheatgrass, Nettle Leaf, Shavegrass, Alfalfa Leaf Juice, Dandelion Leaf Juice, Kamut Grass Juice, Barley Grass Juice, Oat Grass Juice, Burdock Root, Broccoli Juice, Kale Juice, Spinach Juice, Parsley Juice, Carob Pod, Ginger Root, Nopal Cactus, Alma Berry, Spirulina plus an array of other amazing nutrients

What'Supp?

I am not a massive fan of supplements, in many cases you cannot get better than what nature has to offer. However, in a world of over-farming, suspect soil in many regions, and not always the highest quality fruits and veg making their way onto our juicy table, adding the odd supp isn't a bad move. I must make it clear here that if you live near a good local organic farm, chances are you will get everything you need in the soil with which it grows. I only recommend supps if you don't have this luxury.

One thing I am definitely not a fan of though, is vitamin and mineral tablets. They are synthetic and nine times out of ten you simply end up with very expensive wee! I advocate food supps. These are not synthetic pills, but dried real foods, loaded with a plethora of nutrients often not found anywhere else. Take a look around this page and see some of the added nutrition to be gained by adding a little of these amazing supps every now and then to your smoothies. Some, like Spirulina for example, contains 58 times more iron than spinach and 10 times more calcium than milk.

See what adding a small teaspoon of some of these can do for you.

Often you can take a fruit based smoothie and transform it to the next nutritional level by simply adding a teaspoon of a good supp. I highly recommend the Berry Boost, and nearly every time I make a fruit smoothie, a little spoonful of this unique combination of some of the world's finest nutritional berries.

I have developed my own range, as you can see, but there are loads of great quality powders out there. I just like to know exactly what is in my supps and I like to know it's of the highest quality. So you may pay a little more, but the old adage of "you get what you pay for" is never truer than when it comes to food! Like I say, you can get things like wheatgrass and spirulina powder from most good health food stores, so you don't have to buy my brand, I'm just letting you know these are the supps I truly believe in and can really help if you have nutrient deficiencies.

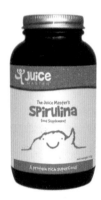

Spirulina

The world's highest beta-carotene content food, and 60% pure protein – making it the most concentrated protein source on earth! Spirulina is claimed to be the only known dietary source of glycogen.
10 x more calcium than milk.
58 × more iron than spinach.
Rich in essential fatty acids.
Rich in easy to absorb iron (not just any old iron you understand).
Rich in vitamin B12.

Wheatgrass Powder

A source of 93 of the 103 minerals required by the human body.

Contains 20 amino acids

11 × more calcium than cow's milk

5 × more iron than spinach

4 × the vitamin B1 of whole-wheat flour

7 × the vitamin C of oranges.

A good source of the elusive vitamin B12.

An excellent source of vitamins C, E, K and B complex.

Rich in calcium, cobalt, iron, magnesium, phosphorus, potassium, sodium, sulphur, and zinc.

Rich in chlorophyll.

See the next page for more information.

Berry Boost

Contains some of the finest berries in the world – which aren't always easy to get hold of. Add a teaspoon to any fruit smoothie to take it to another nutritional level! Look what's in it: blueberry juice, acai, goji berry, pomegranate, bilberry juice, black cherry juice, graviola, black elder berry, saw palmetto berry, hawthorne berry, acerola berry juice.

Detox Boost

Amazing for you, but best not added to a juice as it will make it taste, well – *pants!* Best mixed with a bit of apple juice and taken as a shot!

Wheatgerm

Add a small teaspoon to any fruit smoothie for extra nutrition and an increase in stamina. Wheatgerm oil has been known to increase stamina because of its octacosanol content, a lipid that stimulates the production of androgens and muscle growth.

Ultimate Super Food

There are greens; and then there's **Juice Master's Ultimate Super Food greens**! Contains an incredibly rich array of land vegetables, grasses, spirulina and chlorella, aquatic vegetables, digestive enzymes and probiotics.

Udo's oil

Dr Udo is the "daddy" when it comes to essential oils!

Udo's Choice delivers a reliable source of the omega 3 and omega 6 essential fatty acids that are essential to life – it's a natural source of undamaged EFAs.

High Potency Friendly Bacteria

A unique probiotic formula containing soil-based organisms. These easy-to-swallow capsules provide all the nutrients needed to support a healthy bowel, digestive and immune system.

Hemp Protein Powder

Is a plant based source of 21 amino acids (the building blocks of protein)

Shelled hemp seed or hemp nut contains 51% pure digestible protein, providing readily available amino acids for building and repairing tissue. Hemp seed protein is comprised of 65% high quality edestin protein, the most potent protein of any plant source and 35% globulin edestin, which closely resembles the globulin in blood plasma and is highly compatible with the human digestive system.

Wheatgrass

Cows Eat It, Dopes Smoke It, But only The Enlightened Drink It!

No other juice on earth comes close to the nutritional power of wheatgrass. Just a single shot (30 ml / 1 fl oz) of wheatgrass, in terms of vitamins and minerals, is said to be equivalent to 1 kg (2¼ lb) of other vegetables. There are many ways to get your daily shot, choose the best way for you and get some of this rightly named Super Juice Shot down you every single day.

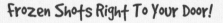

Frozen Shots Right To Your Door!

It is official; there is a God! In the UK a company in Northamptonshire which grows wheatgrass, juices it for you, freezes it into 1 fl oz shots and delivers to your door next day! Yes no juicing, no growing, no cleaning – all done! Visit **www.livewheatgrass.co.uk** and enter the code "jasonvale" and you'll get an extra week of wheatgrass totally free!

It's field-grown wheatgrass and isn't as sweet as some tray-grown grasses, but it's how grass was designed to be grown. And if you follow my little "Tip For Taste" (see facing page) you won't taste a thing.

You Can Even Stick It Up Your Backside!

Yes if you are feeling that way inclined, you can indeed have wheatgrass implants (enemas). They are actually great for healing and detoxifying the colon walls. The implants also heal and cleanse the internal organs. After an enema, wait 20 minutes, then implant 4 ounces of wheatgrass juice. Retain for 20 minutes. If that's just one step too far and your bottom has a strict "No Entry" sign on it - then just drinking the juice will be good enough :)

Wheatgrass Powder

An easy way to get wheatgrass into your system is by using wheatgrass powder. You can get wheatgrass powder in so many places now, but make sure you do your research on the quality!

All you do is either add a teaspoon to a smoothie or you can make a quick shot. This can be done by adding the powder to either water or apple juice (I'd go with the apple juice where possible). To get rid of any powder residue, you can either give it a quick blend, using a hand blender, or add some apple juice to a Protein Shaker, add the powder and shake 'til smooth...*ish*.

The nutritional quality of powdered wheatgrass will never be as good as the freshly extracted juice, but it's still remarkably good, plus it's super convenient so chances are you'll have it more often.

Wheatgrass Highlights

20 amino acids
(including all the essential ones)

11 x more calcium than cow's milk

5 x more iron than spinach

4 x the vitamin B1 of whole-wheat flour

7 x the vitamin C of oranges.

A source of the elusive vitamin B12

A shot of wheatgrass contains more protein than beef.

Excellent source of vitamins C, E, K, B complex.

Rich in calcium, cobalt, iron, magnesium, phosphorus, potassium, sodium, sulphur, and zinc.

Rich in chlorophyll

Fresh Wheatgrass Shot

The best quality wheatgrass juice you can get is when you cut it from freshly grown, and juice it there and then. This of course has its challenges – you have to grow it, cut it, juice it and clean the machine. However, if you have a serious illness, especially the big "C", you need the proper fresh stuff.

One way to make it easier is to find a company that will deliver freshly grown wheatgrass already grown in trays. If not, growing it yourself isn't actually that hard. You can get a growing kit from our site, which takes about 10 days to grow and works out much cheaper than buying a shot at a trendy juice bar in London.

You will also need a masticating juicer. If you already have a good centrifugal juicer, I would recommend getting either a manual wheatgrass juicer or getting just a single gear masticating juicer. Check the wheatgrass page on **www.juicemaster.com** for lots more info as space is tight here!

Tip for Taste

Wheatgrass juice may be very, very good but let's face it, the taste isn't always going to get you doing cartwheels in the snow! So here's a tip: have a slice of orange ready. Drink your shot in one hit (30 ml) and immediately bite into the orange. The orange is good too as it's vitamin C content will help to utilize more of the iron in wheatgrass. So a total win! I never, ever have a shot without a slice of orange near by if I can ever help it – it makes it easy to take rather than – well, you'll see.

Juicy Tips

Apple **Mainly for juicing, but at times you can add a little to your blender** as part of a smoothie. There is no need to peel — a lot of goodness is found in the skin. And there is no need to chop or remove the seeds either. If you have a wide–chute juicer that can fit a whole apple — feel free to do just that!

The harder the apple, the more juice you will get. If you have a two speed juicer, apples should be juiced on the faster speed.

Apple is a great base and sweetens vegetable juices. Mostly use Golden Delicious or Royal Gala. Avoid bitter apples, like Granny Smith, they are just too tart.

Apricot **Can be juiced or smoothied** (made up word). Either way you will need to remove the seed: simply cut down the centre and the seed usually just pops out. If you have a nice ripe one, you can open it with your fingers. Soft very ripe apricots are good for blending as part of a smoothie and hard ones are better in the juicer. As ever, when juicing "soft" fruits set your juicer to its slowest speed.

Asparagus **Juice** (sparingly). This green juice is very potent, so you only need a little — which is a good job as this veg isn't exactly cheap! Always mixed with other juices.

Avocado **Never juice, always blend**! And they must be ripe! Cut in half, remove the stone, scoop out the flesh, and add to a blender with some other juice. Avocados make a creamy smoothie when ripe, but it's not always easy to get them ripe. When you do find some, buy a load and freeze them. Clearly don't freeze as they are – take the flesh and put in suitable container for freezing. You will then have gorgeous ripe avocados whenever you need them.

Banana **Bananas do not juice!** Actually they don't do much at all — they just tend to sit around ;-) Always put bananas in the blender. And make sure they are ripe or they will make your smoothie lumpy! Obviously, remember to remove the skin first! If you buy too many, then simply peel, cut into chunks, and freeze in a suitable container. You then have nice cold bananas to add to your smoothie whenever you please.

Beetroot (or **Beets** if from *US-of-A*) **always juice**, and only *ever* juice **raw** beetroot. Leave the skin on and juice the bulbs as they are. One of the finest sweet juices on earth.

Bell Pepper **Juice for best results**. Simply chop them for the size of your juicer's chute and juice. Beautiful sweet tasting juice.

Berries (all kinds) **Can be juiced or smoothied** – whether blue, black, cran, rasp, straw, etc. An exception is that some berries cannot be juiced from frozen. Berries are usually quite expensive, so I tend to bung them in the blender. If you do juice them, pack them in tight before turning the juicer on – the tighter you pack 'em the more juice you get! And use the juicers slowest speed.

Broccoli **Always juice**. Look for long stems when buying (they are often cheaper as no one else wants them). The stems are loaded with minerals but moreover, you will get the most juice from the stem. You can also juice the florets, but the stems are better.

Cabbage *Cut into chunks and juice*. Always mix with another juice (like apple) as it sucks by itself!

Carrot *Simply juice* – no need to peel. Carrots are one of the finest nutrient-packed ingredients the world has to offer and are a great base for many of the recipes in the book.

Celery *Always juice* – it's far too stringy for your blender! No prep needed here, just juice. Again tastes better when mixed with things like apple juice.

Cherries *Best juiced, but can be smoothied*. Remove the seeds before juicing. Pack into the juicer as tight as possible, and then juice on the slower speed.

Coconut To get the milk from the nut (be careful with this one!): Using a pointed knife or skewer, gently press the three indents on the top until you find the one that will "give". Push through this indent to create a hole. Now you can pour out the milk or perhaps stick a straw in and drink it as it is.

Cranberries (see berries).

Cucumber *Best juiced,* although you can chop into small chunks and add to your blender too, but nearly all recipes in this book require you to simply juice them.

Fennel *Simply cut and juice*. Preparation couldn't be easier! This juice tastes like liquorice – nice!

Garlic *Remove the paper skin and juice*. Please use very sparingly. Garlic juice is very powerful and essential if you have parasites making you sick. I use this in one recipe and one shot in this book (see "Super Shots" – p. 250) but I recommend you don't experiment yourself with this natural antibiotic.

Ginger Root *Juice only and do not peel*. Ginger features heavily throughout this book and for good reason, as you will read in our little facts throughout. The Ginger Shot is also something I recommend you have every single day.

Grapefruit One of the few fruits you must *peel before juicing*. When removing the peel make sure you keep the pith as a great deal of the nutrients are found here and it helps to make the juice deliciously creamy.

Grapes *Best juiced*. You can simply put a bunch of grapes into your juicer, pack them tight to get more juice (making sure machine is OFF first) and juice on speed 1.

Kiwifruit *Juice or smoothie*, your shout! If juicing, simply juice with skin on – very easy! Or, if you wish to add to a smoothie, peel, chop in half and add to the blender.

Lime *Can be juiced with the peel*, so always buy "wax-free" where possible. Some of the recipes in this book ask for you to peel first. This is only for taste as with the skin left on it can make some recipes a little too zesty!

Lemon *Can be juiced with the skin on*, so like limes, if possible buy "wax-free". Lemons feature heavily throughout this book due to their nutritional value and how wonderful they are in adding a kick to a juice. The "World Famous Lemon...Aid" is a prime example of what the humble lemon can do on the taste front. When juicing with the skin on, push through your juicer slowly – so you don't muck up the motor!

Mango *Can be juiced or smoothied*. Either way you will have to remove the large pit (or stone) that runs through this gorgeous fruit. Place the mango on its side, put your knife just to left or right of centre and cut down. You will avoid the stone that way. Simply scoop the flesh from the "bowl" that is left and juice or add to a blender to make smoothie.

Mango juice is very, *very* thick and you will need to dilute with another juice or plenty of ice.

Melon (apart from watermelons) *Should be juiced without the skin*. Simply remove the flesh and juice, no need to remove seeds first, your juicer will simply chuck them into the pulp.

Orange *You must peel before juicing*, as the oils in the skin of oranges are indigestible to humans. When you do, leave as much of the white pith as possible – most of the nutrients are found there and it makes the juice taste creamy. You really have never tasted fresh orange juice until you have juiced one with the pith on!

Parsley *Juice only*. As this is an herb, you need very little. Pack into the juicer tight before you turn the machine on for best juicing results.

Parsnip *Juice only*. No prep needed, keep the peel on and simply juice.

Papaya *Can be juiced or smoothied*. Remove the skin and simply juice or cut into chunks and add to a blender with some juice to make a smoothie. Paw Paw juice isn't really that nice by itself and always needs a little sweetener, such as pineapple juice.

Peach *Best juiced but can go into a blender in chunks* and mixed with juice to make a smoothie. Simply cut open, remove the pit and juice. Peach juice is quite thick so mix it with another juice or plenty of ice.

Pear *Simply juice* with the skin on. Pears juice best when they are quite hard as you get more juice. Conference pears juice very well and are very common. You *could* chop pears and add them into a blender to make a smoothie, but I always juice them.

Pepper (see "Bell Peppers")

Pineapple *Can be juiced or smoothied*. Depending on your juicer you can keep the skin on, however, you will get a smoother juice if you remove the skin before juicing. Pineapple can also go in the blender, but makes the smoothie very stringy, so not always recommended. It helps if the pineapple chunks are frozen if you do this.

Raspberries (see "Berries").

Spinach *Best juiced*. The best way to juice spinach is to pack the leaves into your juicer tight. Make sure the juicer is off when you do this – you don't want to juice your fingers! The tighter you pack the leaves the more juice you will get.

Strawberries (see "Berries").

Clementine / Mandarin / Satsuma / Tangerine Not a great deal of difference between these fruits other than some are easier to peel than others. **All must be peeled before juicing**. Satsumas are very easy to peel, juice really quickly and make a great substitute for orange juice.

Tomato Simply pop them as they are into your juicer.

Turnip *Juice only*. No prep, just juice it on the faster speed. Turnip juice needs to be mixed with something like apple juice to make it palatable. It's worth knowing no other juice matches turnip for it's calcium content.

Watermelon *Can be juiced with the skin on*. No need to remove seeds first, your juicer will simply chuck them out with the pulp.

Wheatgrass *Always juice*. You cannot juice wheatgrass with a normal centrifugal juicer – you will need a masticating juicer (see "Your Funky Fresh Kitchen – p. 14).

Wheatgrass juice should be taken in small "shots" of no more than 2 fl oz at a time. (See What'Supp – p. 252) for more details.

Juicy Measurements

Almost all the measurements in this book are metric. That keeps everything nice and consistent, although I realize that if you're a traditionalist (or from the US of A) you may not be familiar with these measures. Not to worry. When recipes call for a 1 cm or 2 cm chunk of something, you don't need to be too exact. Just estimate it!

2.5 cm = 1 inch

1 small handful = ⅓ cup

1 large handful = ½ cup

240 ml = 1 cup

1 teaspoon (tsp) = approx 5 ml

1 tablespoon (Tbsp) = 3 teaspoons (approx 15 ml)

And just in case, here's a ruler!

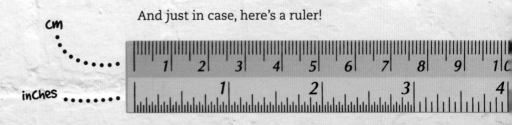

Juicing The World...

Why not help spread the word?

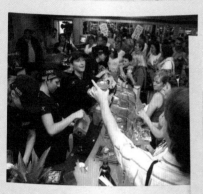

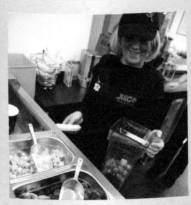

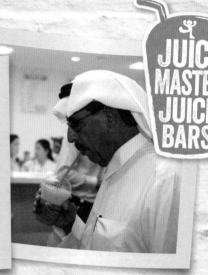

JUICE MASTER JUICE BARS

Juice Master juice bars... currently in Ireland, Dubai, Scotland, China and Canada.

Juice School – We have trained juice therapists all over the world – why not become a Natural Juice Therapist yourself?

Juicing Apps – we even hit number one!

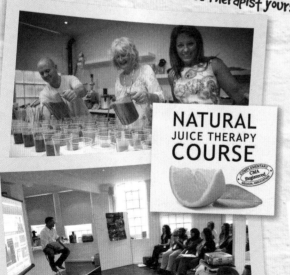

NATURAL JUICE THERAPY COURSE

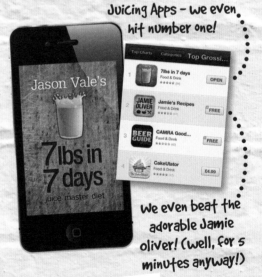

Jason Vale's

7 lbs in 7 days

juice master diet

We even beat the adorable Jamie Oliver! (well, for 5 minutes anyway!)

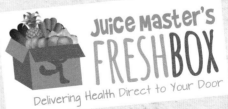

Juice Master's FRESHBOX

Delivering Health Direct to Your Door

We've scoured the UK to find you the best produce for the Juice Master 3, 5 or 7 day detox and we'll deliver it to your door. Juicing has never been easier.

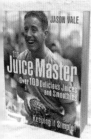
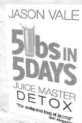
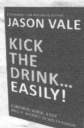
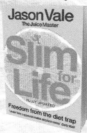
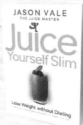
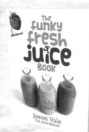

Here are some of the books I've written. If you have a real foodie issue, then I'd get this one.

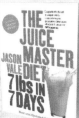
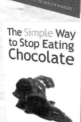

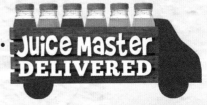

You can now get your juice detox delivered to your door with our new juice delivery service.

Juice Master's very own healthy food bars, a great alternative to other sugary, unhealthy snacks.

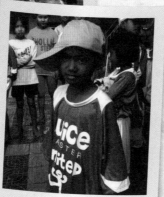
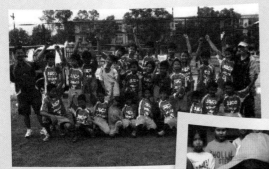

We even sponsor an orphanage in Cambodia – Come on United!

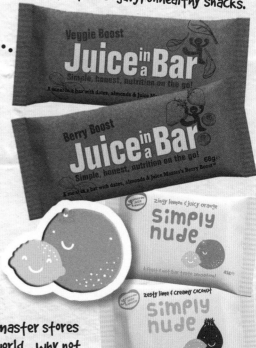

online juice master stores around the world... why not open one in your country?

free downloads and health and juicing info – all available on the site

www.juicemaster.com

Juicy Mountain
Juicing, Yoga & Fitness Retreat
TURKEY

"One of the best weeks of my life..."
- Beverley Knight

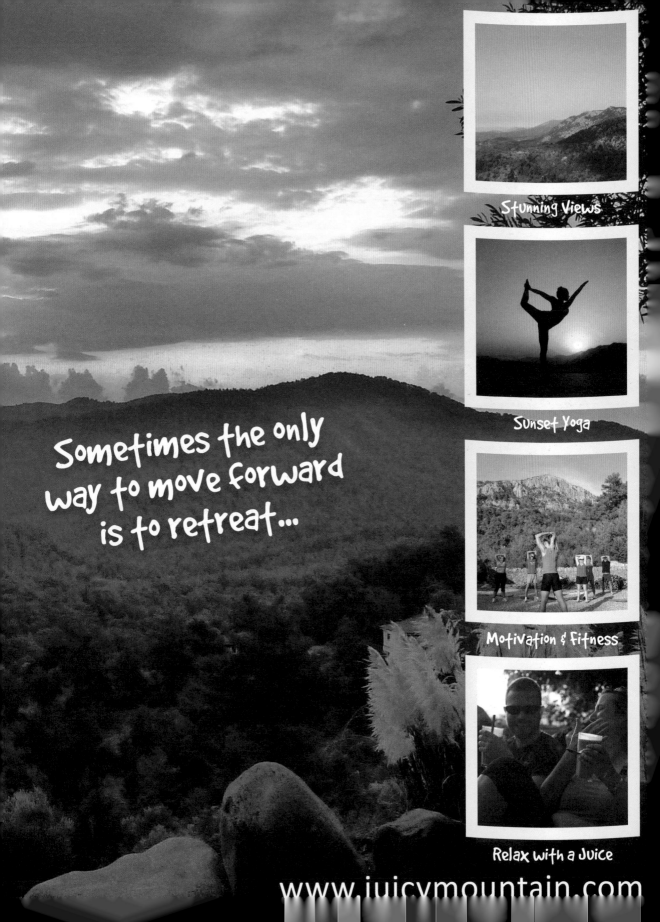

Sometimes the only way to move forward is to retreat...

Stunning Views

Sunset Yoga

Motivation & Fitness

Relax with a Juice

www.juicymountain.com

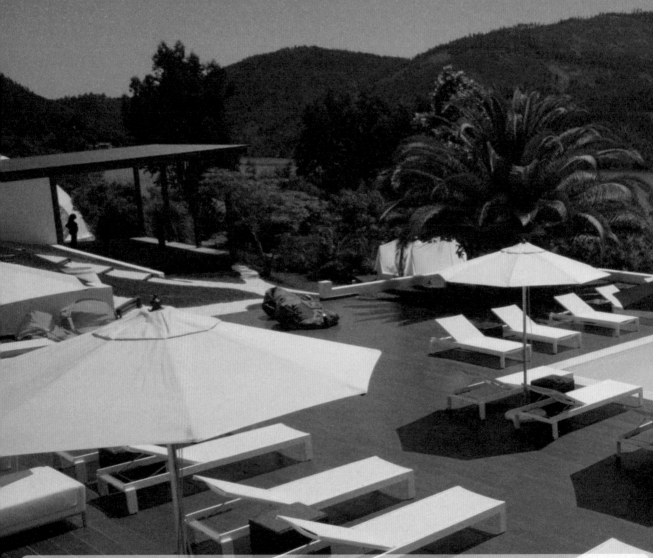
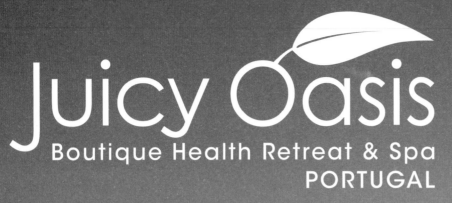

Juicy Oasis
Boutique Health Retreat & Spa
PORTUGAL

"Words can not express how wonderful this place is! But one word that comes to mind is *MAGICAL.*"

- Alesha Dixon

"Life is not measured in the number of breaths we take but by the moments that take our breath away."
Hilary Cooper

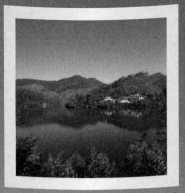
Idyllic Location

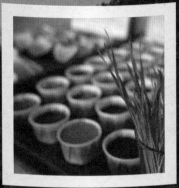
Delicious Juices

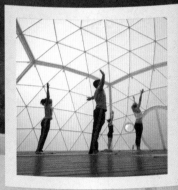
Yoga & Fitness

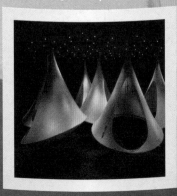
Boutique Spa Experience

www.juicyoasis.com

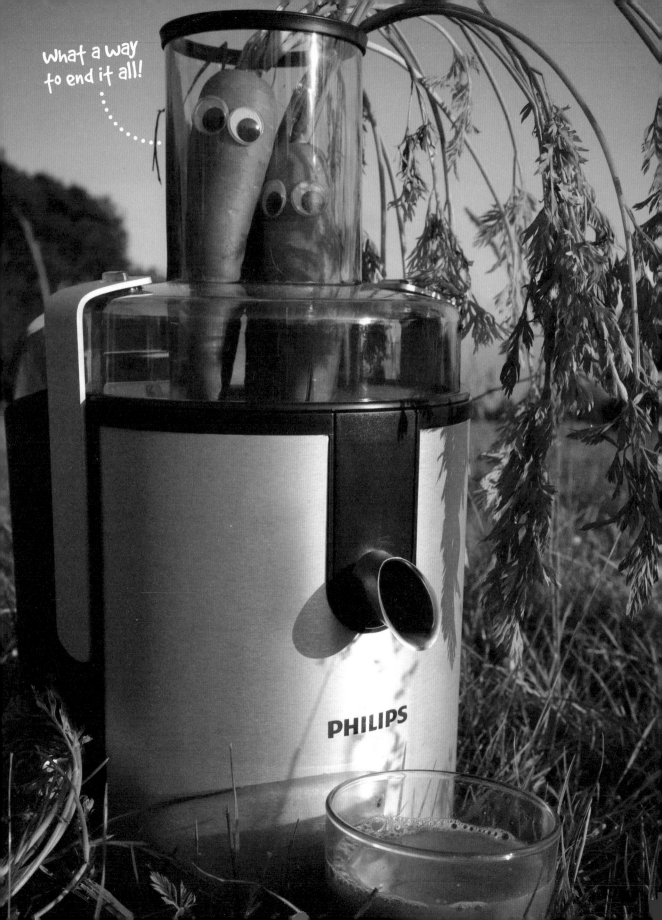